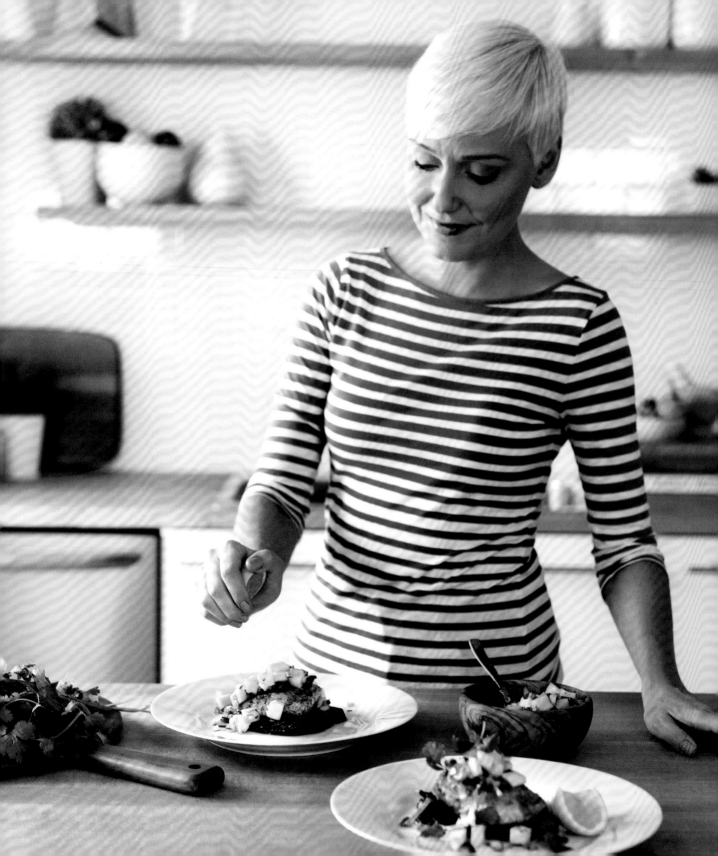

THE
domestic
GEEK'S

MEALS MADE EASY

A Fresh, Fuss-Free Approach to Healthy Cooking

SARA LYNN CAUCHON

WITHDRAWN

HOUGHTON MIFFLIN HARCOURT
BOSTON   NEW YORK   2019

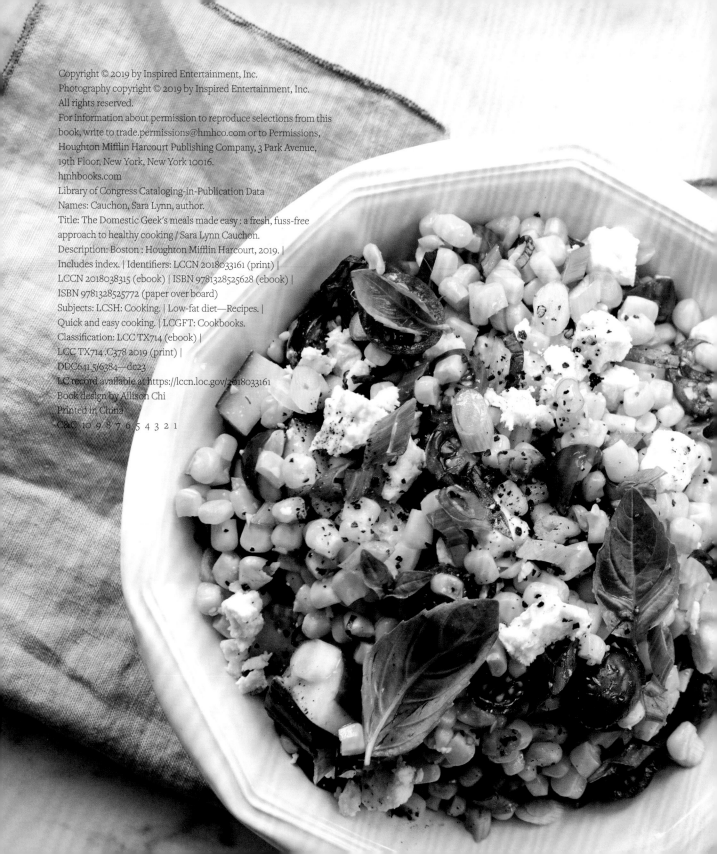

For information about permission to reproduce selections from this
book, write to trade.permissions@hmhco.com or to Permissions,
Houghton Mifflin Harcourt Publishing Company, 3 Park Avenue,
19th Floor, New York, New York 10016.

hmhbooks.com

Library of Congress Cataloging-in-Publication Data
Names: Cauchon, Sara Lynn, author.
Title: The Domestic Geek's meals made easy : a fresh, fuss-free
approach to healthy cooking / Sara Lynn Cauchon.
Description: Boston : Houghton Mifflin Harcourt, 2019. |
Includes index. | Identifiers: LCCN 2018033161 (print) |
LCCN 2018038315 (ebook) | ISBN 9781328525628 (ebook) |
ISBN 9781328525772 (paper over board)
Subjects: LCSH: Cooking. | Low-fat diet—Recipes. |
Quick and easy cooking. | LCGFT: Cookbooks.
Classification: LCC TX714 (ebook) |
LCC TX714 .C378 2019 (print) |
DDC 641.5/6384—dc23
LC record available at https://lccn.loc.gov/2018033161

Book design by Allison Chi
Printed in China
C&C 10 9 8 7 6 5 4 3 2 1

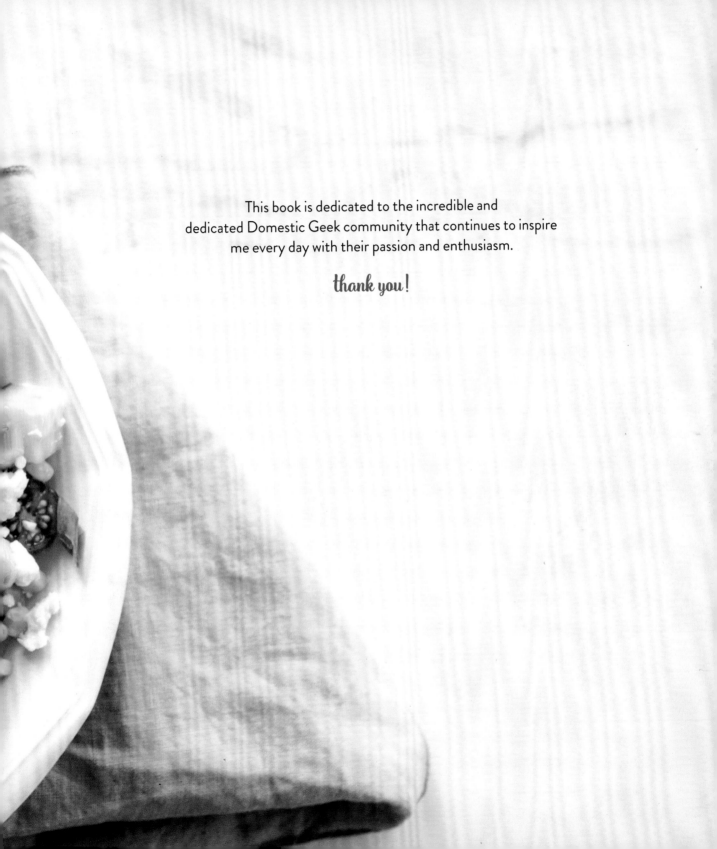

This book is dedicated to the incredible and
dedicated Domestic Geek community that continues to inspire
me every day with their passion and enthusiasm.

thank you!

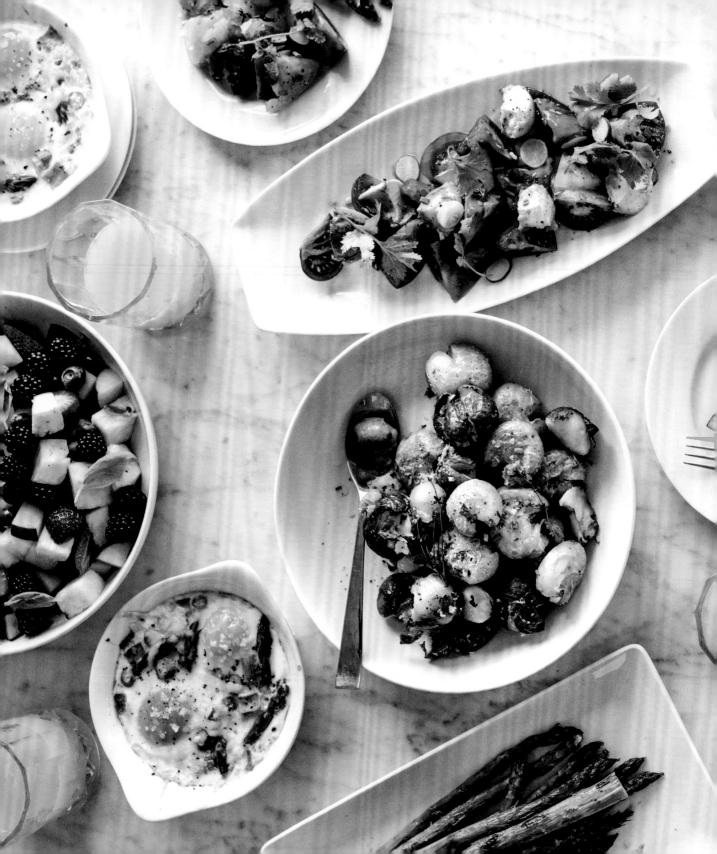

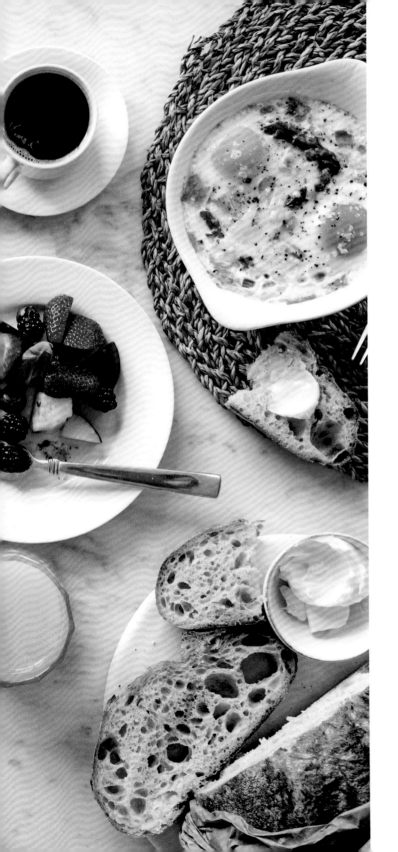

contents

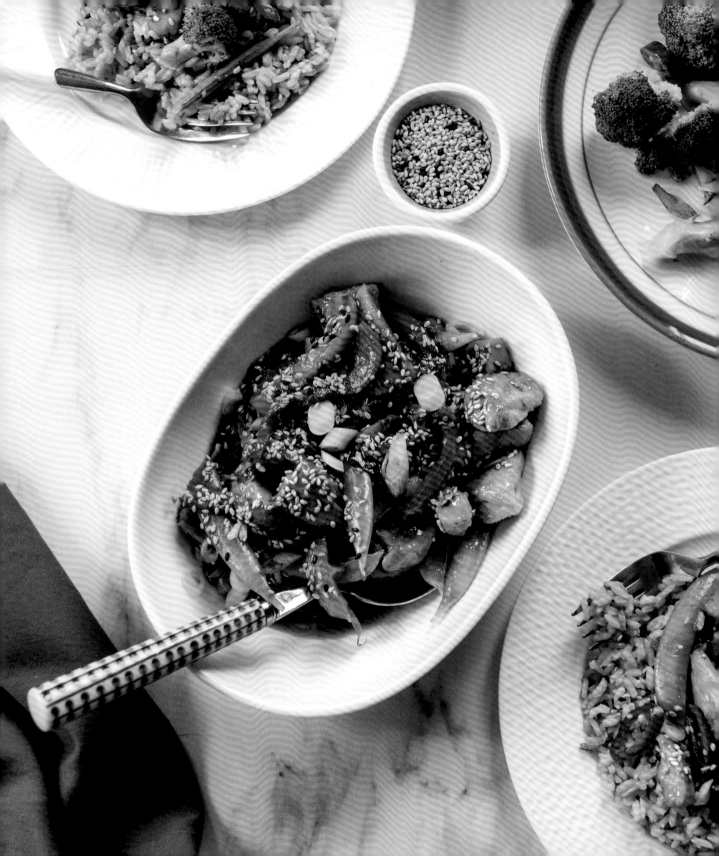

acknowledgments

I CAN honestly say that when I started on this journey, I really had no idea what I was getting into. Writing a cookbook is so different from running a food blog or creating YouTube videos, but is something that I have wanted to do for as long as I can remember. This book has truly been a labor of love, and I am so very grateful to the incredibly supportive and inspiring people who helped me bring it to life.

First and foremost, I have to thank my business partner and "work wife," Sarah Bolen, for her patience and constant encouragement through this process. She always gives me lots of creative freedom but also knows how to gently keep me on track when I get obsessive—which happens from time to time.

I also want to extend a major thanks to my amazing colleague Alisa Furniss, who worked in the kitchen for months to ensure that each and every one of these recipes was tested until perfect. I couldn't have done this without her. And also to the rest of the Domestic Geek team—Casey Jones and Emily Purcell—who remain so dedicated to creating delicious content for our incredible online community. I couldn't ask for a more talented and kind group of people to work with every day.

When it comes to a cookbook, mouthwatering food photography is a must, and I wouldn't have trusted this project to anyone but my dear friend Kyla Zanardi, who is both wildly talented and extremely patient, and helped me bring this vision to life. I also want to thank our amazing styling team—Dara Sutin, Houston Mausner, and Rayna Schwartz—who, with seemingly no effort at all, makes everything look more delicious than I could ever even imagine.

And then there's the book itself, which would have never come to be without the gentle nudging of my amazing agent, Samantha Haywood, who somehow believed I could do this before I ever did. And of course, I want to extend my sincerest appreciation to our publishers, Justin Schwartz and Andrea Magyar, who have been huge champions of this project from the very beginning. Thanks to you both for guiding me through this unfamiliar and intimidating process and for working so collaboratively with me to see it to fruition.

And finally, I want to send a huge thanks to my amazing family that has loved me every step of the way and remains the Domestic Geek's biggest cheerleaders all these years later. Especially my husband, Gregory, who stood by me when I decided to quit my full-time job as a television producer to become a YouTube creator, and who didn't complain when I took over our tiny kitchen and then our entire house to make this dream a reality, and who continues to believe, even today, that I am capable of achieving anything I can imagine. xo

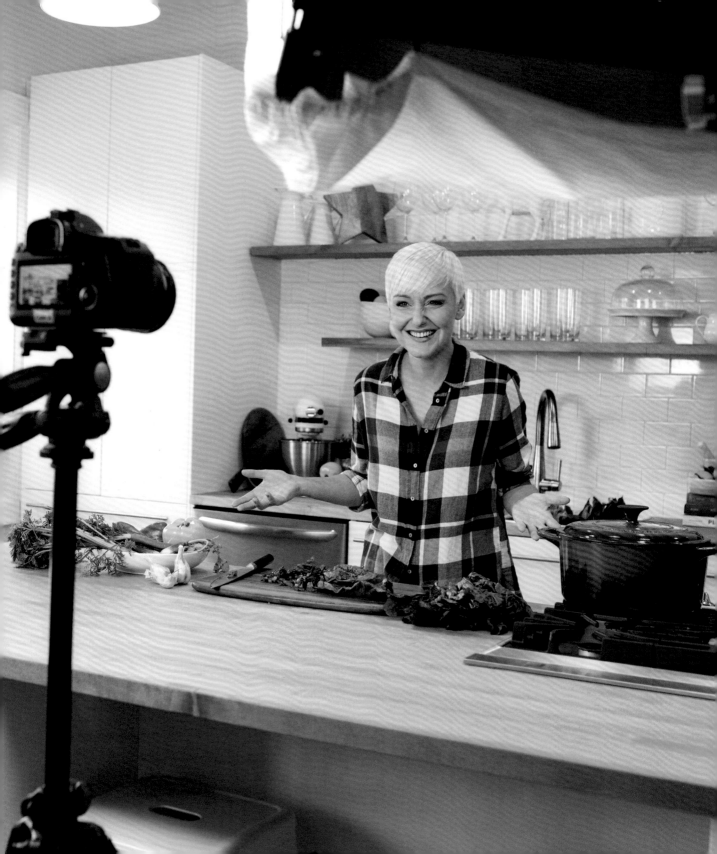

introduction

HI THERE! I'm guessing that if you're reading this, you want to eat better; that healthy eating is important to you and that you want to do more of it. But also that you're busy—working, studying, generally being awesome—and what little time you do have, you don't necessarily want to spend in the kitchen. I get it. That's why my goal is to make eating well easier. Oh, and a lot more delicious, of course.

In my experience, the secret is not fancy ingredients, tools, or techniques. It's about having a collection of simple recipes that can be prepared quickly, affordably, and, above all, *easily*, but that you also actually want to eat. I hope this book is just that.

I'm Sara Lynn, by the way, and if you're new to the Domestic Geek community, WELCOME! I've spent the last five years dishing out all sorts of deliciousness on YouTube, Facebook, Instagram, and just about anywhere else hungry people seek kitchen inspiration. It's amazing to think that in that time, our cooking collective has grown to include more than 1.5 million dedicated food enthusiasts. A total dream come true, especially for someone who adores all things edible as much as I do.

Food was really my first love. Growing up, cooking was always my favorite thing to do. While other kids were watching cartoons or cheesy sitcoms, I was watching cooking shows and then heading into the kitchen to test newly discovered recipes and techniques. My parents were always incredibly supportive and, as parents do, politely choked down anything I served up with a spirited "Good job!" whether it was particularly palatable or not. (Thanks, Mom and Dad!)

But it wasn't enough for me to just cook the recipes, oh no. Channeling my beloved TV chefs, I would talk my imaginary audience through each and every step, recommending a pinch of this or a splash of that to a plethora of endlessly attentive stuffed animals. (Who, in retrospect, were probably grateful for their lack of hearing—and taste buds, for that matter.)

As I grew up, my tastes grew with me, and I spent my early twenties experimenting with all sorts of exotic flavors and fussy French techniques. I traveled all over on eating adventures and discovered so many new cuisines along the way. I was so obsessed, in fact, that every week my fellow foodies and I hosted a Friday night supper club, where we'd try daring new recipes over too many bottles of wine.

And like good wine, my cooking skills improved with age, but the amount of time I spent in the kitchen became less and less. As a busy professional, I just didn't have endless hours to stand at the stove anymore, and most often found myself either eating out or ordering in—habits that were jeopardizing both my health and my bank account. Something needed to change, so back to the kitchen I went.

I learned to meal plan and committed to Sunday meal prep—a few hours dedicated to shopping, prepping, and cooking foods to enjoy through the week. You probably won't be surprised to hear that my health began to improve almost immediately. I had more energy and better digestion, and I started to see the weight that had snuck up on me thanks to years of take-out start to vanish. I wasn't doing anything really extraordinary, but the impact of just eating at home was simply incredible. The most dramatic improvement, though, was my confidence, and I couldn't wait to share that feeling with the world.

I launched *The Domestic Geek* in April 2014 to inspire others to eat well and as a result, live better, with a fresh, fuss-free approach to healthy cooking. The objective since its inception has always been to make life in the kitchen easier, which is why *Meals Made Easy* felt like such a fitting title for this collection of recipes that aims to do just that. I hope you enjoy them!

WHAT DOES
"healthy" even mean?

WE'RE BOMBARDED with the word *healthy* every day—in news articles, blog posts, billboards, pop-up ads, and cookbooks all claiming they have the key to longer lives and smaller waists. Even the institutions we really trust can't define it. Researchers are divided, evidence is conflicting, and, let's be honest, "facts" aren't what they used to be. It's easy to feel like the word has really lost all meaning, if it ever really had any to begin with.

The truth is that "healthy" is totally subjective and means something different to each of us. But whether you count carbs, calories, macros, or minutes until your next meal, what I know for sure is that you probably want to be eating better, and I'm here to help with that. And while I certainly can't define healthy as it relates to the rest of the world, I can share what it means to me and what it means in the context of this book.

Healthy begins with whole foods; like the kind you find at the local farmers' market or around the perimeter of your grocery store—bright, vibrant, fresh ingredients that spark your imagination and inspire you to get into the kitchen to create something amazing.

Healthy means cooking and eating at home. (Almost) anything you make at home is going to be better for you than something you picked up at a fastfood joint or had delivered. Let's admit it—take-out is taking a serious toll on our waistlines, our wallets, and our well-being. Just making our own food gives us back control over what we're putting into our bodies and that's half the battle.

Healthy means balance. I could have easily written a book all about kale or quinoa or chia seeds (all of which are great, by the way), but I can totally admit that while I love those superfoods, I also have a pretty strong affinity for more indulgent ingredients like freshly grated Parmesan cheese and good-quality sourdough bread. I also happen to enjoy butter—quite a bit, actually—so everything in moderation, right?

Healthy means satiating. You can eat all the salad you want, but if you're still starving when you're finished, you haven't done yourself any favors. Food is meant to nourish the body and the soul, so healthy should also mean hearty and filling and comforting. It doesn't necessarily mean feeling stuffed, but it definitely means feeling satisfied.

And I'm sure you have your own definition of what healthy means, so while I hope you find this book inspiring, I also hope you'll take these recipes and make them your very own. Try them, test them, and tweak them until they're just right for you. After all, healthy also means making your health and yourself a priority.

essentials

IN THE next few sections, I'll share some of my kitchen must-haves. If you're already an advanced cook or you're just really hungry, feel free to skip right ahead to the Recipe section on page 32 where the deliciousness begins. But if you're looking to maximize efficiency and minimize effort when you cook, you might find these essentials helpful along the way.

KITCHEN ESSENTIALS

I learned to cook in a very small kitchen where there just wasn't a lot of room for silly gadgets or extra appliances that only did one job. That's why, when it comes to stocking a kitchen, I am all about the basics. You probably already have a lot of these items in your own kitchen, but if not, most of them can be purchased inexpensively at your local big-box store. These will all come in handy as you work your way through the recipes in this book.

MIXING BOWLS

A set of mixing bowls is invaluable in the kitchen. Glass is always good, but metal bowls are generally more affordable and, of course, more durable. You'll want a small bowl for prepping things like sauces and vinaigrettes, a medium bowl for mixing up baked goods, and a large bowl for jobs like tossing the perfect salad (like the irresistible Creamy Greek Pasta Salad on page 99).

MEASURING CUPS AND SPOONS

Now, I'll admit, I'm terrible at measuring things when I'm cooking. A dash of this and a splash of that is usually how I roll. That being said, if you're a beginner cook,

you'll likely find measuring tools really useful when making these recipes. And while cooking is mostly an art, where improvisation is encouraged, baking is most definitely science, so using proper measurements is critical when making something like the Chocolate Chia Breakfast Cookies on page 40.

SILICONE (RUBBER) SPATULA

I probably have a dozen rubber spatulas in all shapes, sizes, and colors in my kitchen. Because they're very flexible, they're great for getting that last drop of honey out of the measuring cup. And because they're made of a soft, pliable material, you can use them in your nonstick pans without scratching the finish. They're really affordable, so I recommend picking up two or three in different sizes, if you can.

WHISK

A good metal whisk is the very best tool for beating eggs or mixing up flavorful vinaigrettes like the ones on pages 224 through 227. I have a big whisk and a little whisk, but both do basically the same job.

COLANDER

My metal colander gets a ton of use in my kitchen. I use it to wash fruits and vegetables, to drain and rinse canned beans, and of course for straining cooked pasta. I fancy a metal colander over a plastic one, but it's really just a matter of personal preference. If you can spring for a large colander *and* a smaller one, that's even better.

CUTTING BOARDS

You'll notice that I've made this plural. Every kitchen needs two cutting boards—one for produce and one for meat and fish. I use two different-colored boards so I don't get them mixed up. Both plastic and wooden boards are great, but I suggest avoiding glass or marble boards because they're very unkind to your knives. I prefer to use dishwasher-safe boards that can be sanitized in very hot water.

KNIVES

If you're ever going to splurge on a kitchen tool, your chef's knife is definitely the place to do it. A good-quality chef's knife is the single most important tool in your arsenal and will actually make your life in the kitchen much easier and much more enjoyable. Since good knives can run anywhere from $50 to $200, I recommend asking for one as a birthday or Christmas gift. The good news is that a good-quality knife will last for years, as long as it's sharpened regularly and cared for properly. Other knives that are great to have on hand are a paring knife, a filet knife, and a serrated bread knife.

SMALL SAUCEPAN WITH A LID

A small saucepan (about 2 quarts) is so useful for cooking up rice, quinoa, or even boiling eggs. This little pot doesn't have to be pricey to be really valuable in the kitchen. I also love it for making single servings of oatmeal or reheating leftovers if you don't have a microwave.

HIGH-SIDED SKILLET WITH A LID

When it comes to pots and pans, a high-sided skillet is probably the most versatile one you'll find. You can simmer, sauté, and stir-fry in them effortlessly. And if you spend a little more on a nonstick version that's also oven-safe, it's probably the only pan you'll really ever need. I always recommend purchasing one with a tight-fitting lid, which will allow you to use it to steam ingredients as well. Use it to cook up the delicious Balsamic-Glazed Chicken on page 135, or to give the Turkey Taco Quinoa Skillet on page 128 a try.

DUTCH OVEN

If you've ever watched my YouTube videos, you probably know that I am OBSESSED with my Dutch oven. It's the perfect choice for soups, stews, and the One-Pot Pastas you'll find on pages 159 to 162. It's also amazing because it's oven-safe. Keep in mind that Dutch ovens can really range in price. They can be as low as $50 or run as high as $350. Mine was only $60 and I've had it for nearly ten years. I'm not convinced that the more expensive ones are really any better, so I recommend purchasing one on the lower end.

BAKING SHEETS (SHEET PANS)

I always recommend having at least two baking sheets on hand. They should have rolled sides that are about ¾ inch high. Be careful not to use the flat cookie sheets with no edges (for anything other than cookies, of course), because those can lead to major messes in the oven. Obviously baking sheets are great for tasks like baking and roasting, but I actually use them to make entire meals like the incredible Sheet Pan Suppers on pages 148 to 152. If you don't have nonstick baking sheets, do yourself a favor and line them with parchment paper before you get cooking. Trust me, it will save you so much time and energy when it comes to doing the dishes.

MEAT THERMOMETER

If you don't have one already, I implore you to put this right at the top of your must-have list. You'll quickly notice that when it comes to recipes in this book that involve whole cuts of meat or poultry, I will always include a safe internal temperature reference. To be clear, there is *no* safer way to tell if a cut of meat is properly cooked than with a meat thermometer. There are both analog and digital versions available, and they can cost as little as $10 or as much as $100, but no matter what you pay, you'll never regret this investment. Plus, how else will you know when the strip loin for your delicious Steak Salad with Warm Tomato Vinaigrette (page 140) is the perfect medium-rare?

RASP-STYLE GRATER

A rasp-style grater is the best tool for grating ingredients like garlic, ginger, and Parmesan cheese as well as zesting citrus fruits like lemons, limes, and oranges. You might say it's a "grate inzestment." Sorry, sometimes I simply can't resist a good food pun (or two, for that matter). Rasp graters can be found in lots of different sizes, but I prefer one that's wider across since it's more versatile. The major brands can be quite pricey, but there are great no-name versions that are just as effective and a lot more affordable.

CITRUS PRESS

This might not constitute a must-have but it certainly is a nice-to-have, especially when you love citrus fruit as much as I do. A citrus press is the best tool for getting maximum juice from your lemons and limes; plus, you don't have to worry about those pesky seeds sneaking into your dish, which is a real bonus. This handy-dandy kitchen accessory is ideal when making the fresh salsas featured on pages 214 to 217 or the lemony Healthy Chicken Piccata on page 131.

JULIENNE PEELER

As someone who has always struggled with limited counter space, a spiralizer just isn't very realistic, so I prefer to use a simple julienne peeler, which kind of looks like a traditional vegetable peeler but has little "teeth" that can julienne vegetables like carrots, cucumbers, and zucchini. You'll find this tool particularly handy if you're making the delicious Fresh Rainbow Rolls on page 124 or the tangy Pad Thai Zoodles on page 156.

BLENDER

As you may already know, smoothies are kind of my jam. In fact, I've probably shared more than one hundred smoothie recipes since I first launched my YouTube channel. (I've shared a few of my very favorites on pages 72 through 76, so be sure to take a look!) And as a bit of a smoothie connoisseur, I'll tell you that you don't need a fancy-schmancy blender to get your smoothie on. The blender I use today was less than $100 and works just fine. If you want to splurge on a $500 blender, you're welcome to, of course, but I don't think it's absolutely necessary.

FOOD PROCESSOR

I *love* my food processor, as you'll probably notice when you start sifting through the pages of this book. Once again, you don't have to spend big money on a very high-end model, but to make life in the kitchen easier, a food processor is a must. How else are you going to try the rich, creamy Classic Hummus on page 221? And keep in mind that most food processors come with extra attachments that are great for slicing, shredding, and more.

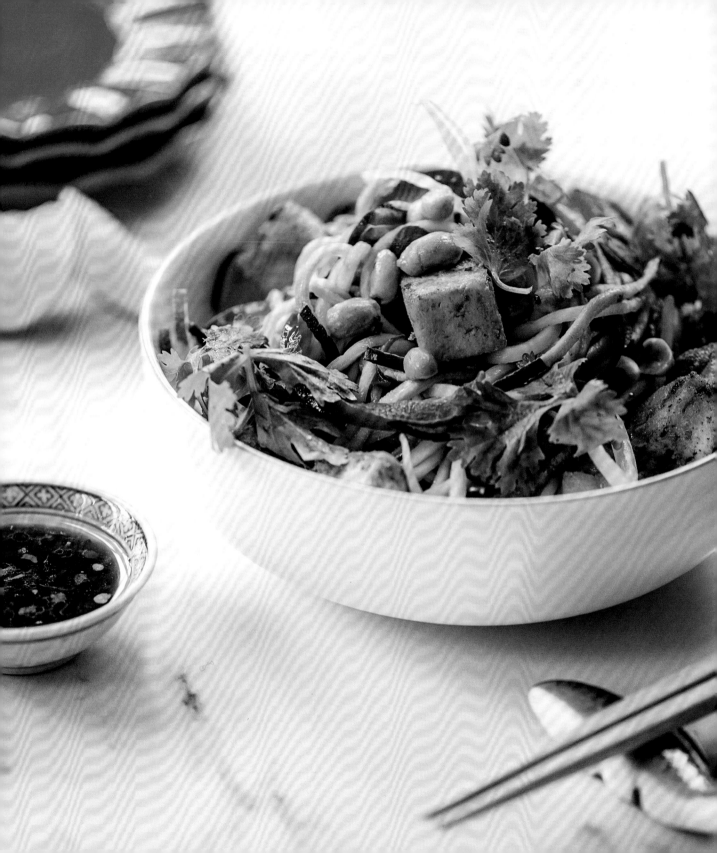

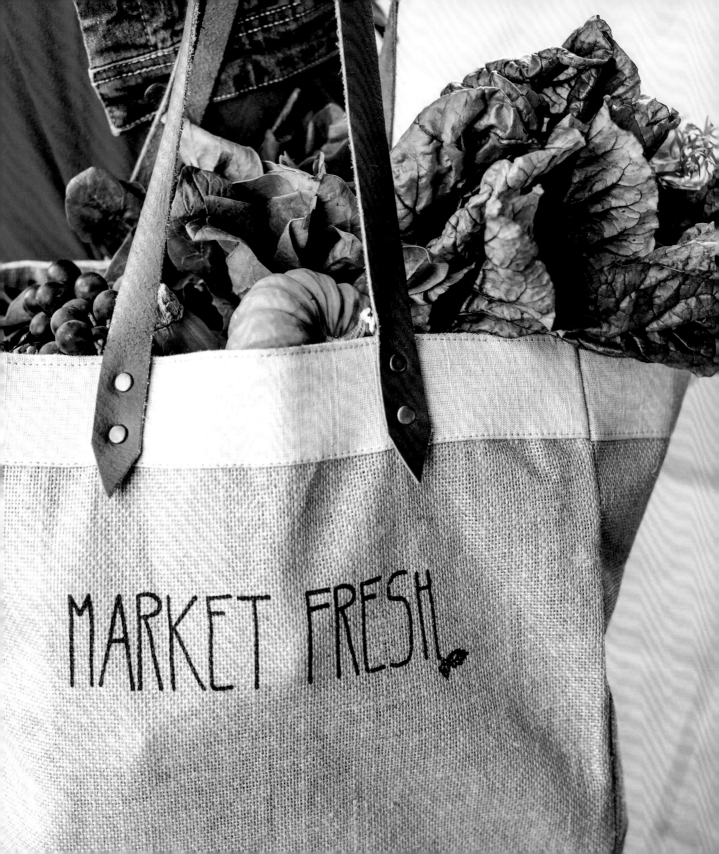

FRESH ESSENTIALS

I think the real secret to eating well is filling your fridge with food that you actually want to eat. Buy produce that is vibrant and colorful so you know you're getting a variety of vitamins and minerals, but also so it looks lush and appealing and makes you want to take a bite. Buy local produce, eggs, dairy, and meat when and if you can. The closer to home your food is raised or grown, the better. Buy organic if it's available and affordable. Consider your food's impact not just on your own health but also on the health of the world around you. Above all, buy fresh food that motivates you to get into the kitchen and cook.

FRESH VEGETABLES

Love them or loathe them, vegetables are the foundation for any healthy, balanced diet. When selecting your vegetables for the week, use the rainbow as your inspiration. Start with bright leafy greens like romaine and kale. Then add crisp cruciferous veggies like broccoli or Brussels sprouts. Top up with ruby reds like tomatoes and bell peppers and vibrant oranges like carrots and sweet potatoes, and round it out with sunny sweet corn and deep purple cabbage. Even if you're not a big vegetable lover, identify one in each color that you can enjoy, and start with those.

FRESH FRUIT

Fresh fruit is, understandably, almost always easier to swallow than vegetables. Most people I know adore fresh fruit and with good reason—it's packed with nutrients that your body craves, and it also happens to taste really good. Bright berries, tart citrus, mellow melon—I suggest loading up on them all. But just be aware that with all that delicious fruit also comes a lot of sugar. And even though it's natural sugar, like anything, it should be enjoyed in moderation.

EGGS

In my humble opinion, there is no food more perfect than eggs. They're packed with protein, vitamins, and minerals and take mere minutes to prepare. In fact, I think eggs are actually the *easiest* food to make, and there are countless ways to enjoy them. I always recommend buying local, organic eggs if possible. Store them in the refrigerator, of course, but avoid putting them in the door because that's where the most temperature fluctuations happen, and you want your eggs to be kept consistently cold. If you're vegan, many of the recipes in this book that call for eggs can be modified to use a "flax egg" instead. To make a flax egg, mix 1 tablespoon ground flaxseed with 2 tablespoons water and let it sit for 10 minutes to gel. I've indicated where a flax egg can be used in the Simple Swaps section.

MILK

Milk remains an absolute staple ingredient in so much of my cooking, but there are many options beyond dairy available now. In this book, I've primarily used 2% milk, but that can easily be substituted in most cases with the milk of your choice. If you're using dairy milk, you can certainly swap out the 2% for whole or skim. If you prefer to go dairy-free, almost all the milk in these recipes can be substituted for unsweetened almond, cashew, soy, or rice milk.

GREEK YOGURT

Greek yogurt is both protein-packed and probiotic-rich, which has elevated it to superfood status. I prefer to purchase plain Greek yogurt, since most flavored yogurts contain a ton of additional sugar. I also opt for the full-fat version whenever possible. Good fat, like the kind found in natural yogurt, helps keep you feeling fuller longer, which I love, and low-fat yogurt often contains unnecessary additives that I'm happy to live without. Of course, Greek yogurt can be enjoyed all on its own, but I like to use it as a substitute for mayo in things like chicken salad or as a topping in place of sour cream. I even use it in my baking—see my Good Morning Muffins on page 54.

CHEESE

I'll admit it—I'm a cheese addict. It's true. My mom was a deli manager when I was growing up, so our fridge was always full of cheese of every variety. But while I absolutely adore it, cheese moderation is essential. When buying cheese, I always skip the low-fat stuff and spring for the best quality I can afford. When it comes to shredded cheese, I recommend grating it yourself instead of buying the pre-shredded, pre-packaged kind. Not only will you save some cash, you'll also be avoiding lots of additives.

Many of my recipes call for freshly grated Parmesan cheese. Parmesan is one place that I am an absolute purist, so please avoid the canned version you find in the grocery aisle. I know that Parmesan can be pricey, so I always buy a big chunk when I find it on sale. And remember that good Parmesan is so flavorful that a little goes a very long way, so it will last you a while. Keep in mind that Parmesan cheese is made with animal rennet, so it is not considered vegetarian.

Finally, if you don't eat dairy, there are lots of great cheese alternatives on the market now that are definitely worth a try, and more are popping up all the time.

BUTTER

Yes, I said butter. While any fat should be consumed with moderation in mind, butter is not necessarily bad for us, as was once believed. It's much less processed than its competitors and even contains essential vitamins and minerals. Not to mention the fact that it tastes pretty wonderful smeared on a slice of crusty French bread. Compared to other cooking fats, butter imparts more flavor in a dish and adds a richness that's hard to duplicate. That said, if you don't consume dairy, there are several excellent butter substitutes on the market now, with more on the way.

PANTRY ESSENTIALS

While I love having my fridge filled with lots of fresh food, it's equally important to keep a well-stocked pantry. Keeping these items topped up will ensure you always have an answer when asked, "What's for dinner?" or breakfast and lunch, for that matter.

OATS

Old-fashioned rolled oats are an absolute staple, especially when it comes to breakfast. They're loaded with protein and fiber, so they're great for your health and can be prepared in a million different ways. I love using them in my crisp Homemade Granola on pages 63 to 65, my chewy and delicious Baked Oatmeal Cups on page 32, and my great-on-the-go Overnight Oatmeal on page 44. And if you're only eating oats for breakfast, you're definitely missing out. They can also be ground up as a substitute for flour in your baking, used as a replacement for bread crumbs in meat loaf and burgers, or even turned into a savory side dish with a splash of chicken broth and some sautéed veggies—yum! Keep in mind that while old-fashioned oats are naturally gluten-free, they are sometimes processed in facilities where they can come into contact with wheat products. If avoiding wheat products is important to you, look for "gluten-free" on the packaging.

RICE

Rice is used in almost every cuisine around the world, and it's really no wonder! It's affordable, easy to prepare, and has such a neutral flavor that it can be paired with almost anything. I always have white, brown, and long-grain and wild rice on hand so I can switch things up and keep it interesting. If you're looking to maximize your rice's potential, pair it with fiber-rich beans—the combination creates a complete protein source and a seriously delicious dish. If you're looking for a little inspiration, I highly recommend the incredible Cajun Rice & Beans on page 155.

QUINOA

If you're skeptical about quinoa, you're not alone. There are lots of folks out there who struggle with its unusual texture and nutty flavor. That being said, the health benefits of this superfood simply can't be under-estimated. It's packed with plant-based protein and enough fiber to keep you full, so I always have some stocked in the pantry. I recommend buying it in bulk and only when it's on sale, since it can be pretty pricey. And if you're just used to eating it plain, you're missing out on a world of flavor possibilities. I definitely rec-ommend trying the Tangy Thai Quinoa on page 80, the subtly sweet Berry Almond Quinoa on page 34, or my all-time favorite Veggie Fried Quinoa on page 112.

DRIED PASTA

Pasta has gotten a bad rap over the past few years, but I believe there's still a place for it on the dinner table—in moderation, of course. Pasta is quick, easy, and inex-pensive, making it a godsend on a busy weeknight. And if you start preparing One-Pot Pastas like the ones on pages 159 to 162, even washing the dishes will be less time-consuming. I always have some penne, rotini, spaghetti, and fettuccine in my pantry, but really, any shape will do. And if you're concerned about your glu-ten consumption, most supermarkets now carry lots of corn-, rice-, or quinoa-based wheat-free pastas.

CANNED DICED TOMATOES

Growing up, my mother put canned diced tomatoes in basically everything because they were versatile but also really inexpensive. So now, as an adult, of course I buy them by the case. Adding diced tomatoes to a soup, stew, chili, or pasta instantly infuses the dish with a rich heartiness that is just so satisfying. Plus, they're packed with flavor without being packed with calories. What's not to love about that? You'll find them in my to-die-for Turkey Taco Quinoa Skillet on page 128 and my smoky Chipotle Chicken Chili on page 141.

CANNED BLACK BEANS

Beans, beans, the musical fruit, the more you eat, the more you . . . oh, never mind! My pantry would feel naked without a can or two of black beans stocked inside. In fact, I am so obsessed with this fiber-rich, protein-packed legume that, like diced tomatoes, I usually buy them by the case. Because of their neutral flavor, they can be added to so many different dishes. They're great when cooked with rice or added to chili or even stuffed into sweet potatoes, but I think their best quality is that they can even be enjoyed cold in a dish like my zesty Southwestern Black Bean Salad (page 89).

CANNED CHICKPEAS

Chickpeas (also known as garbanzo beans) are another protein powerhouse that can be used in countless dishes. Like black beans, I prefer to buy them canned instead of dried because they're much more convenient to cook with and can be enjoyed almost instantly. I always recommend rinsing your chickpeas and beans before using them to wash off any additional salt. Try them in the vegetarian Falafel Burger on page 154 or the almost-too-good-to-be-true Chickpea & Avocado Smash Sandwich on page 100.

TUNA

Canned tuna is one of the most convenient sources of protein you can find, so it's always a good idea to have some in the cupboard. Try to find sustainable brands if you can, and always buy the kind without any added salt. Trust me, we're all probably getting enough salt in our lives as it is. And if you've only ever had tuna spread on a sandwich, your taste buds are in for a real treat, because the Mediterranean Tuna Salad on page 122 will blow you away!

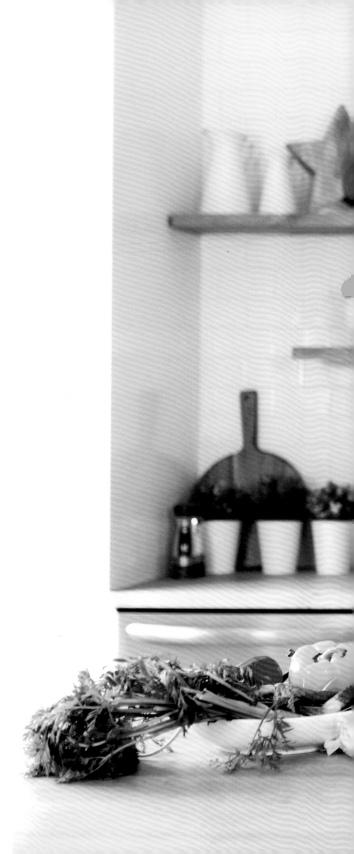

BROTH

When it comes to broth, nothing beats homemade (try my recipe on page 204), but in a pinch, having some store-bought broth tucked away in the pantry is always good planning. Chicken, beef, mushroom, vegetable . . . you really can't go wrong. In fact, I would say I use broth more than any other ingredient in my cooking. Obviously it's the base for most great soups and stews, but it's also amazing for cooking things like rice or quinoa or for deglazing a pan or turning drippings into some tasty gravy. The list really goes on and on. In this book, broth is just about everywhere, but if you really want to taste it at its best, I would suggest trying my ooey-gooey, irresistible Classic French Onion Soup (page 175).

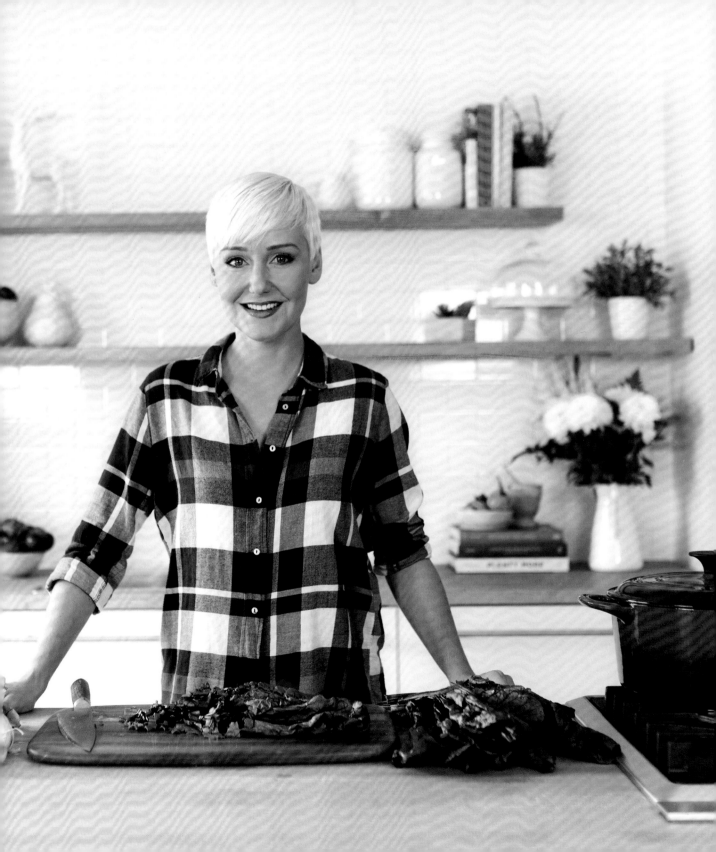

cooking
MADE EASY

ABOVE ALL, this book was written to help make your life in the kitchen easier. Here are a few tips for simplifying the cooking process that I've always found extremely helpful . . .

MISE EN PLACE

Practicing the French art of *mise en place* will basically change your life in the kitchen. The concept of *mise en place*, which simply translates to "put in place," is to gather and prepare all your ingredients (and your cooking tools) before you start cooking. This includes rinsing, chopping, measuring, etc. Once you've got all your ingredients and utensils "put in place," the cooking can begin. Working this way takes a little more time off the top but will inevitably make the cooking process so much smoother and a lot more enjoyable.

USE A SHARP KNIFE

Dull knives are not just inefficient, they can be extremely dangerous as well. A dull knife is more likely to slip and cause an accident than a very sharp one. If you're not comfortable sharpening your knives yourself, you can have them sharpened professionally. It's a small investment but totally worthwhile when you think about how much easier kitchen prep will be. I recommend sharpening your knives two or three times a year, depending on how frequently you cook.

HONE YOUR KNIFE SKILLS

You don't have to chop like a TV chef to get the job done, but learning the proper way to use a knife and chop common fruits and vegetables will ultimately make cooking feel like less of a chore. There are a million free tutorials online to help with this. Search "how to chop an onion" or "the best way to peel a kiwi," and you'll learn so much. In addition, get a better understanding of different chopping techniques. What's the difference between "dice" and "finely dice"? What's julienne? What's chiffonade? Learning these common cuts will make your cooking more efficient.

DON'T RUSH IT

Even easy recipes deserve time to reach their maximum potential, so be patient when you're cooking. You'll notice that when a recipe is made on the stove, I never suggest heating your pan above medium-high, with the exception of boiling water. It's just too easy to burn delicate ingredients and ruin their flavor, so be gentle with your heat, and when in doubt, always go low instead of high.

MEAL PREP

As far as I'm concerned, the single best way to make cooking easier is to commit to a few hours of prep each and every week. Read on for some great ways to maximize your meal prep.

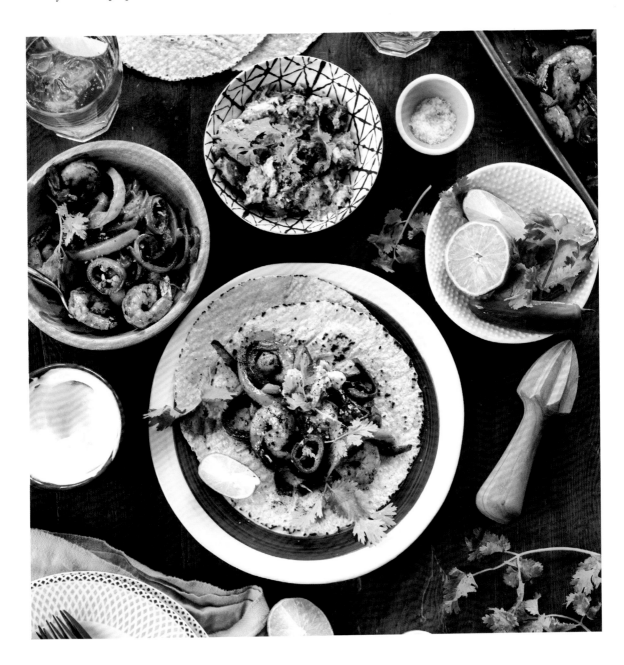

meal prep
MADE EASY

I REALLY believe that Sunday meal prep is the foundation for healthy eating all week long. Spending just a few hours in the kitchen every Sunday can help make cooking so much easier throughout the week, especially when you're tired and so tempted to order take-out.

First off, it should be said that there really is no right or wrong way to meal prep. Some people prefer to do just a little prep like chopping vegetables and washing fruit, while others would rather get an entire week of cooking out of the way in a day. How much you prep in advance is completely up to you, but here are some strategies that I've used to help make my weekly prep a success . . .

PLAN AHEAD
The first step is to write out your weekly meal plan *before* you head to the grocery store. Select the meals you'll be making for the week and create a list of all the ingredients you'll need for those recipes. Then make a list of the ingredients that can be prepared in advance and stored until you need them.

PREP EVERYTHING
When you get home with your groceries, do not put anything in the refrigerator until it has been prepped. That means rinsing your fruit, peeling your veggies, and chopping anything that will be used in recipes throughout the week. Keep in mind that some fruits and vegetables, such as berries and mixed greens, shouldn't be rinsed in advance because they tend to spoil more quickly that way. They should be rinsed just before using.

STORE FOODS SAFELY
Below is a handy guide to help you store foods safely in the refrigerator or freezer once they've been prepped.

	Refrigerator	Freezer
Cooked Meats	3 to 4 days	Up to 3 months
Cooked Poultry	3 to 4 days	Up to 3 months
Cooked Fish & Seafood	2 to 3 days	Up to 3 months
Meat Broth and Gravy	2 to 3 days	Up to 6 months
Eggs, cooked	Up to 5 days	Don't freeze well
Cooked Rice & Quinoa	3 to 4 days	Up to 6 months

my 10 meal prep musts

HERE ARE some foods that I like to prepare each and every week to help keep my eating on track and make weeknight cooking a little easier. You'll also see that these ingredients will be found over and over in recipes throughout this book.

1. BEGIN BY PREPARING SOME PROTEIN. I recommend roasting a whole chicken or a side of salmon to be used in recipes throughout the week. If you're a vegetarian, consider marinating some tofu that can be baked or grilled later.

2. BOIL AND PEEL SOME EGGS. These can be eaten for breakfast on busy mornings or added to salads, like the gorgeous Niçoise Salad on page 85, for lunch.

3. COOK A GRAIN, ANY GRAIN. White rice, brown rice, quinoa (which is technically a seed)—whatever you prefer. Cooked grains are great to add to salads, soups, and chilis, or to serve with dinner.

4. STEAM SOME GREENS FOR THE WEEK. Broccoli, green beans, or asparagus are all great options that are delicious eaten hot or cold. The greens can be added to recipes or served as a side dish.

5. PREP YOUR LEAFY GREENS. Chop them, wash them, and then store them in a zipper bag with a paper towel to keep them fresher longer. This works particularly well with heartier greens like kale, Swiss chard, and romaine lettuce. More delicate greens like baby spinach should be prepped right before eating.

6. PLAN YOUR DINNERS FOR THE WEEK and see if there's any prep work than can be done ahead of time. Chop ingredients like onions, celery, and garlic and store them in airtight containers until you're ready to cook with them. Consider premeasuring ingredients where possible.

7. WASH, PEEL, AND CHOP VEGETABLES FOR SNACKING. I like prepping bell peppers, cucumbers, carrots, and celery and storing them with a healthy dip like the classic Tzatziki Sauce on page 222.

8. RINSE, PEEL, AND CHOP YOUR FRUIT and then divide it into individual servings. This makes it easier to practice good portion control and to enjoy fruit on the go.

9. MAKE SMOOTHIE PACKS by combining your smoothie ingredients in individual zipper bags. These can be stored in the freezer and then blended with milk or juice for an easy breakfast. You can find loads of smoothie inspiration on pages 72 through 77.

10. MIX UP ANY MARINADES, dressings, sauces, or seasoning blends you'll need for your cooking throughout the week.

how to use this book

MIX IT UP

The very best recipes are the kind that can be customized to your personal tastes, so this book is full of great options for pretty much any palate; even the pickiest eaters should find something satisfying. Keep your eyes open for the Mix It Up sections throughout the book. They feature delicious ways to switch up the flavors in a recipe and keep things interesting.

SIMPLE SWAPS

I don't personally subscribe to any particular diet, but I know that a lot of you do, so I've done my best to include lots of great options for all. At the top of each page, you'll see notes that indicate if a recipe is Wheat-Free, Dairy-Free, Pescatarian, Vegetarian, or Vegan, while the Simple Swaps sections provide easy ways to adjust a recipe to complement any dietary preferences.

COOK TIMES

Cook times can vary tremendously and are affected by everything from the type of stove you use to the altitude at which you are cooking (true story!). Every recipe in this book has been triple tested for accuracy, but cook times should always be taken with a grain of salt (pun totally intended). To make things easier, I've included visual cues where possible to help you assess whether something is cooked enough. When it comes to meat though, safety is paramount, and the most accurate way to know if it's cooked properly is to use a meat thermometer.

COOKING OIL

Choosing an oil to cook with is really a matter of preference. For most of these recipes, I like to use a neutral, flavorless oil so the taste doesn't come through in the food. I generally opt for vegetable oil or canola oil in my cooking, but grapeseed, corn, sunflower, and safflower oils are all great options. They all have pros and cons, but none will affect the outcome of the recipe. Coconut oil is also very commonly used now, but can impart a mild coconut flavor, so use your discretion.

I don't typically cook with olive oil unless I'm making a dish with Mediterranean or Middle Eastern flavors. While it has amazing health benefits, it also has a strong taste that tends to come through in a dish, so use it when you know it will complement a dish. I prefer to save it for sauces and yummy vinaigrettes.

When a recipe calls for butter, it's likely because I wanted to add some additional flavor to the dish. If you don't eat butter, simply replace it with a neutral cooking oil like the ones listed above.

SPICE

I am a big fan of spicy foods, so you'll see a lot of red pepper flakes, hot sauce, sriracha, and jalapeños and other chiles in my recipes. These are always optional, so if you're not a fan of heat, you can certainly leave them out without impacting the final dish.

The exception to this is chipotle pepper, which is both spicy *and* smoky. If you're considering removing chipotle from a dish, I always recommend replacing it with 2 teaspoons smoked paprika so you still get the smokiness without the heat.

CILANTRO

Cilantro (or fresh coriander) is a very popular herb in many cuisines around the world. I use it often to garnish dishes because it adds a lot of freshness. That said, there are a lot of folks who do not enjoy the taste of cilantro, and some who downright loathe it. Cilantro is also optional. You can replace it in most recipes with some fresh flat-leaf parsley, or just skip the herbs entirely. The choice is yours.

WHAT IF I DON'T LIKE VEGETABLES?

Believe it or not, this is a question I get asked pretty often. I fully appreciate that lots of people struggle to enjoy the taste of vegetables. Hey, I used to be one of those people myself! But the truth is, there is simply no substitute for fresh vegetables in a healthy, balanced diet, so it's important that we learn to love them (or at least not hate them), and hopefully some of these recipes will help you do that.

I've learned that it's possible to train yourself to enjoy a food by introducing it over and over again until you develop a taste for it. I actually did this with tomatoes, mushrooms, and even with cilantro, which I used to despise. But eating these foods consistently over time helped me develop my palate, and now I can't get enough of them.

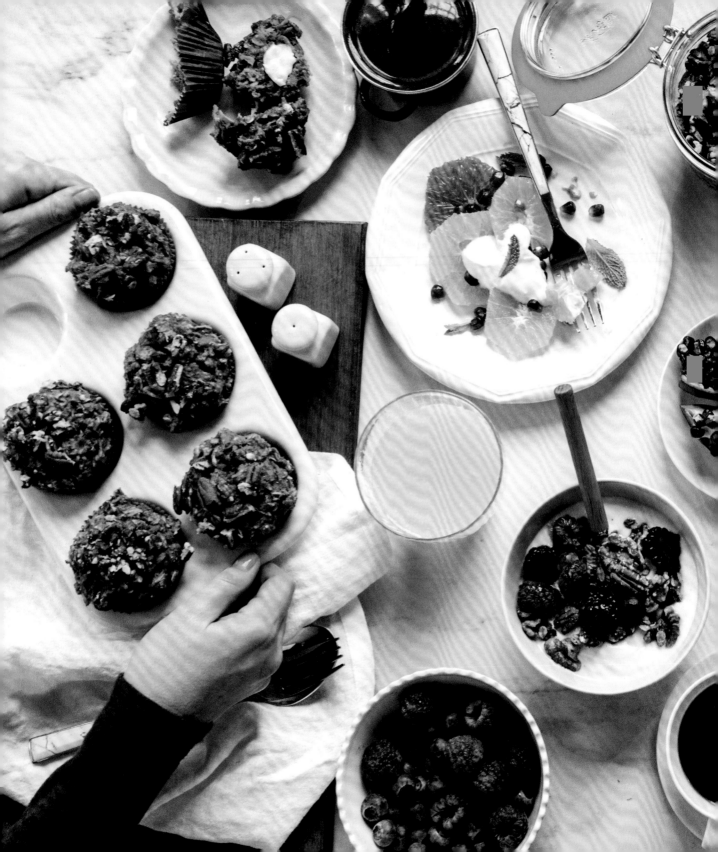

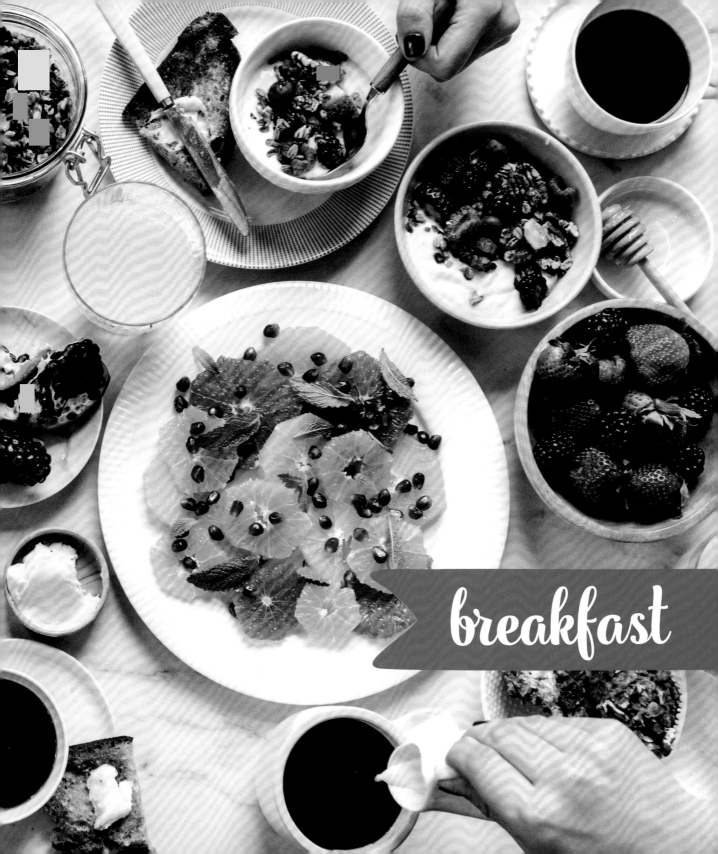

breakfast

BAKED OATMEAL CUPS

VEGETARIAN
WHEAT-FREE
PESCATARIAN

Baked Oatmeal Cups have crisp, golden tops and soft, chewy centers that make them simply irresistible in my house. Just like traditional oatmeal, they are loaded with fiber, which makes them super filling, and baking them individually in a muffin tin elevates them to the perfect grab-and-go breakfast. This classic recipe is lightly sweetened and can be customized with countless tasty add-ins to make it just right for you. These freeze beautifully, so don't be afraid to double or triple the recipe and save some for later—trust me, you won't regret it.

SERVINGS: **12**   PREP TIME: **5 MINUTES**   COOK TIME: **25 TO 30 MINUTES**

Cooking spray (optional)

3 cups old-fashioned rolled oats

½ cup packed light brown sugar

2 teaspoons baking powder

1 cup unsweetened applesauce

1 cup 2% milk

2 large eggs

1 teaspoon vanilla extract

PREHEAT the oven to 375°F. Lightly grease a 12-cup muffin pan with cooking spray or use silicone baking cups.

IN a large bowl, combine the oats, brown sugar, and baking powder. Stir well and set aside. In a second bowl, whisk together the applesauce, milk, eggs, and vanilla. Pour the wet ingredients into the dry ingredients and mix.

SCOOP the batter into the prepared muffin pan. Bake until the muffins are just golden on top, 25 to 30 minutes. Remove the muffins from the pan and let cool for at least 5 minutes.

SERVE warm from the oven or at room temperature, or let cool completely and store in the refrigerator for up to 1 week or in the freezer for up to 6 months.

mix it up

BANANA-BLUEBERRY BAKED OATMEAL CUPS
Swap the applesauce for 3 mashed bananas and fold 1 cup fresh blueberries into the batter before filling the muffin pan.

CHOCOLATE-ALMOND BAKED OATMEAL CUPS
Stir ½ cup semisweet chocolate chips and ½ cup chopped almonds into the batter before filling the muffin pan, to add both sweetness and crunch.

PUMPKIN SPICE BAKED OATMEAL CUPS
Instead of using unsweetened applesauce, add 1 cup pure pumpkin puree and 2 teaspoons Pumpkin Pie Spice (page 231) to the batter. Top each with a whole pecan before baking.

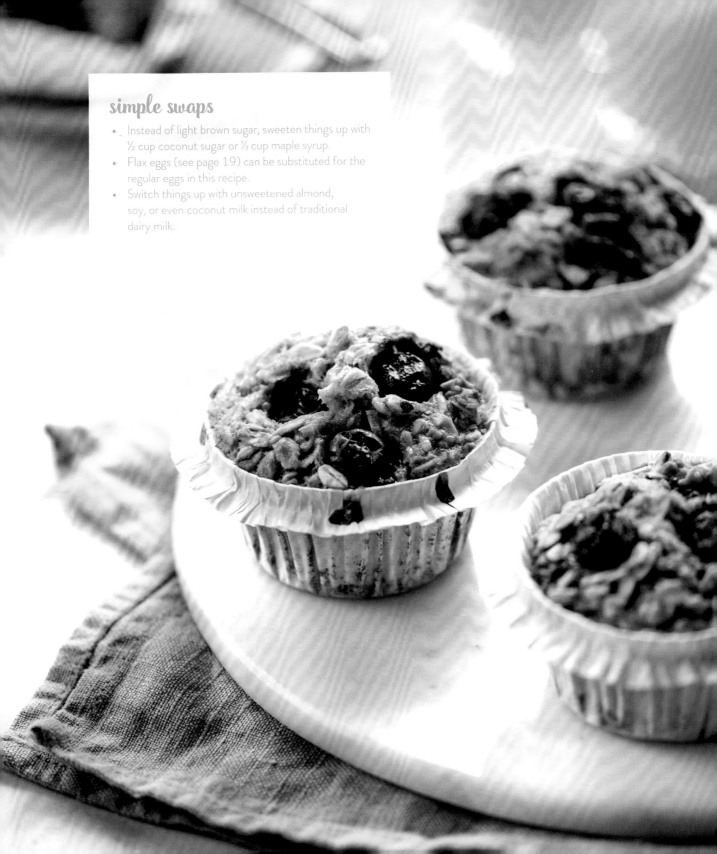

simple swaps

- Instead of light brown sugar, sweeten things up with ½ cup coconut sugar or ⅓ cup maple syrup.
- Flax eggs (see page 19) can be substituted for the regular eggs in this recipe.
- Switch things up with unsweetened almond, soy, or even coconut milk instead of traditional dairy milk.

BERRY ALMOND QUINOA

When it comes to plant-based protein sources, nothing beats quinoa. This super seed contains all the essential amino acids that make up a complete protein, which is why it's so beloved by vegetarians, vegans, and fitness buffs alike. But while most quinoa recipes you'll find tend to be savory, quinoa's natural nutty flavor lends itself beautifully to sweet dishes like my delicious Berry Almond Quinoa, which is perfect for breakfast.

SERVINGS: **4**   PREP TIME: **5 MINUTES**

---

3 cups cooked quinoa (see below)

1 cup quartered strawberries

½ cup blackberries

½ cup blueberries

¼ cup chopped almonds

2 tablespoons maple syrup

IN a large bowl, combine all the ingredients and toss well. Enjoy immediately or cover and store in the refrigerator for up to 4 days.

simple swaps

I use maple syrup in this recipe, but both honey and agave syrup make sweet substitutes.

mix it up
TROPICAL QUINOA
Add a tropical twist to this recipe by swapping the berries for 1 cup chopped pineapple, ½ cup chopped mango, and ½ cup chopped kiwi. Replace the maple syrup with 2 tablespoons honey.

◀ HOW TO COOK QUINOA ▶

COOK TIME: **20 MINUTES**

1 cup quinoa

2 cups water

Combine the quinoa and water in a medium saucepan. Bring the water to a boil over medium-high heat, then reduce the heat to low, cover, and simmer for 15 minutes, or until all the liquid has been absorbed. Fluff the cooked quinoa with a fork before serving. MAKES 3 CUPS COOKED QUINOA

*Quinoa has a natural coating called saponin, which can be slightly bitter. Most of the quinoa you purchase at the supermarket today has already been thoroughly rinsed to remove any bitterness, so there's no need for additional rinsing at home.

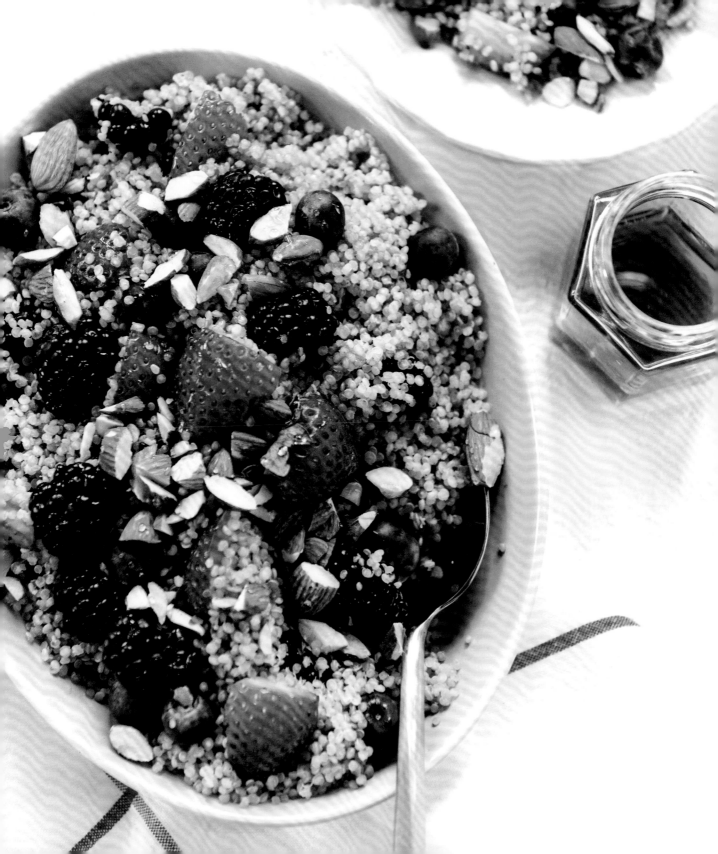

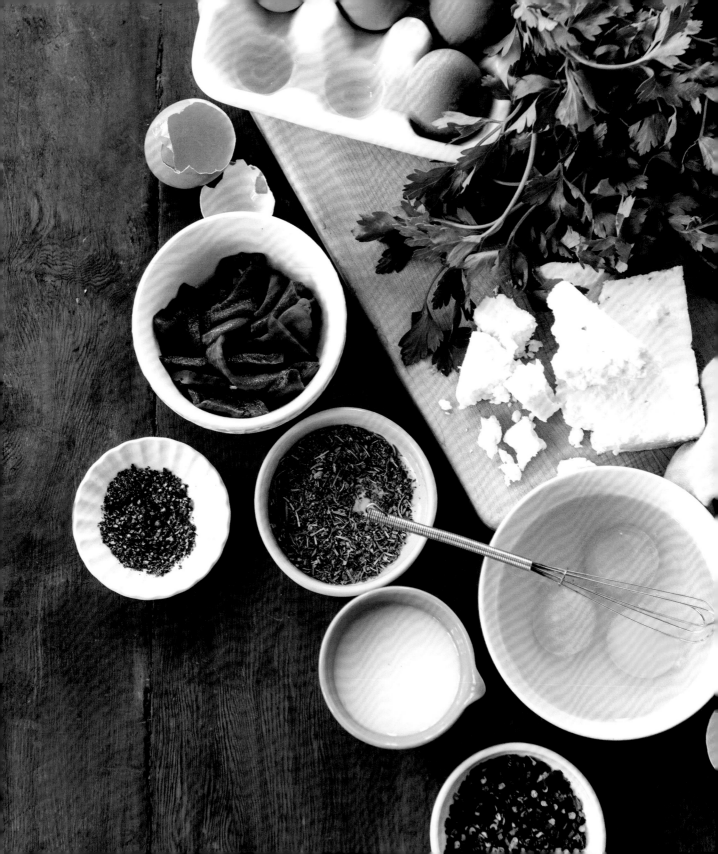

MAKE-AHEAD MINI FRITTATAS

I LOVE eggs for breakfast, but my busy mornings usually don't allow for fussy omelets or oozy eggs Benedict. That's why I simply can't get enough of these Make-Ahead Mini Frittatas! They're protein-packed, gluten-free, and (best of all) portable, so they make eating on-the-go a total breeze. I love to make a big batch during my Sunday meal prep because they'll last up to 4 days in the refrigerator (if you can resist eating them that long).

ROASTED RED PEPPER & FETA FRITTATAS

VEGETARIAN
WHEAT-FREE
PESCATARIAN

SERVINGS: **6**   PREP TIME: **5 MINUTES**   COOK TIME: **20 MINUTES**

Cooking spray (optional)

½ cup chopped roasted red peppers

½ cup crumbled feta cheese

2 tablespoons chopped fresh parsley

6 large eggs

2 tablespoons 2% milk

½ teaspoon Italian Seasoning (page 230)

¼ teaspoon red pepper flakes (optional)

Salt and freshly ground black pepper

PREHEAT the oven to 375°F. Grease a 6-cup muffin pan with cooking spray or use silicone baking cups.

IN a small bowl, combine the roasted red peppers, feta, and parsley. Stir well. Divide the mixture evenly among the prepared muffin cups.

IN a large bowl or measuring cup, whisk together the eggs, milk, Italian Seasoning, red pepper flakes (if using), and salt and pepper. Pour the egg mixture into each muffin cup, leaving just ¼ inch of space at the top.

BAKE for 18 to 20 minutes, until the eggs have completely set and the top is lightly golden.

SERVE immediately or let cool completely and store in the refrigerator for up to 4 days. These mini frittatas can be served cold or reheated in the microwave.

MUSHROOM & SPINACH FRITTATAS

SERVINGS: **6**   PREP TIME: **5 MINUTES**   COOK TIME: **30 MINUTES**

Cooking spray (optional)

1 tablespoon butter

2 cups sliced cremini or white button mushrooms

1 garlic clove, minced

2 cups baby spinach (3 to 4 ounces)

6 large eggs

2 tablespoons 2% milk

Salt and freshly ground black pepper

PREHEAT the oven to 375°F. Grease a 6-cup muffin pan with cooking spray or use silicone baking cups.

IN a large skillet, melt the butter over medium-high heat. Add the mushrooms and cook, stirring often, until they release their moisture and become soft, 6 to 8 minutes. Add the garlic and cook, stirring, for an additional 30 seconds. Add the spinach and cook, stirring, until it wilts, about 3 minutes.

DIVIDE the mushroom mixture among the prepared muffin cups.

IN a large bowl or measuring cup, whisk together the eggs, milk, and salt and pepper. Pour the egg mixture into each muffin cup, leaving just ¼ inch of space at the top.

BAKE for 18 to 20 minutes, until the eggs have completely set and the top is lightly golden.

SERVE immediately or let cool completely and store in the refrigerator for up to 4 days. These mini frittatas can be served cold or reheated in the microwave.

BROCCOLI & CHEDDAR FRITTATAS

SERVINGS: **6**   PREP TIME: **10 MINUTES**   COOK TIME: **25 MINUTES**

Cooking spray (optional)

1 tablespoon butter

½ cup finely diced onion

1 garlic clove, minced

1 cup small broccoli florets

¼ cup water

½ cup grated cheddar cheese

6 large eggs

2 tablespoons 2% milk

Salt and freshly ground black pepper

PREHEAT the oven to 375°F. Grease a 6-cup muffin pan with cooking spray or use silicone baking cups.

IN a large skillet with a tight-fitting lid, melt the butter over medium-high heat. Add the onion and cook, stirring, until translucent, 3 to 4 minutes. Stir in the garlic and cook until fragrant, about 30 seconds. Add the broccoli and water and stir well. Cover and cook until the broccoli begins to soften, 1 to 2 minutes. Remove the lid and allow any remaining water to cook off.

DIVIDE the broccoli mixture evenly among the prepared muffin cups. Top each with 1 tablespoon plus 1 teaspoon of the cheese.

IN a large bowl or measuring cup, whisk together the eggs, milk, and salt and pepper. Pour the egg mixture into each muffin cup, leaving just ¼ inch of space at the top.

BAKE for 18 to 20 minutes, until the eggs have completely set and the top is lightly golden.

SERVE immediately or let cool completely and store in the refrigerator for up to 4 days. These mini frittatas can be served cold or reheated in the microwave.

CHOCOLATE CHIA BREAKFAST COOKIES

VEGETARIAN

VEGAN

WHEAT-FREE

DAIRY-FREE

PESCATARIAN

Yep, you read that correctly . . . Chocolate. Chia. Breakfast. Cookies. Vegan, gluten-free, dairy-free, and absolutely IRRESISTIBLE! Don't believe me? Try them for yourself.

SERVINGS: **12**   PREP TIME: **15 MINUTES**   COOK TIME: **14 MINUTES**

---

2 large ripe bananas

1 cup smooth natural almond butter

¼ cup chia seeds, soaked in ¼ cup water for 10 minutes

¼ cup unsweetened cocoa powder

¼ cup coconut sugar

1 teaspoon vanilla extract

1 teaspoon baking powder

PREHEAT the oven to 350°F. Line a baking sheet with parchment paper.

IN a large bowl, mash the bananas until they are smooth. Add the remaining ingredients and mix until well combined. Spoon heaping tablespoons of the mixture onto the prepared baking sheet.

BAKE for 14 minutes.

LET cool on the baking sheet for 5 minutes before enjoying them. Keep in mind that these cookies are soft, chewy, and have a cake-like texture, as opposed to the crisp cookies you might be used to. You can also let them cool completely and store in the refrigerator for up to 5 days or in the freezer for up to 3 months.

mix it up

These delicious cookies are pretty perfect all on their own but adding some thoughtful mix-ins can make them even more incredible.

CHOCOLATE CHERRY
Fold ⅓ cup dried cherries into the batter before transferring it to the baking sheet.

DOUBLE CHOCOLATE
Fold ⅓ cup vegan dark chocolate chips into the batter before transferring it to the baking sheet.

CHOCOLATE PEANUT BUTTER
Swap the almond butter for 1 cup smooth natural peanut butter and stir ⅓ cup chopped peanuts into the batter (for crunch) before transferring it to the baking sheet.

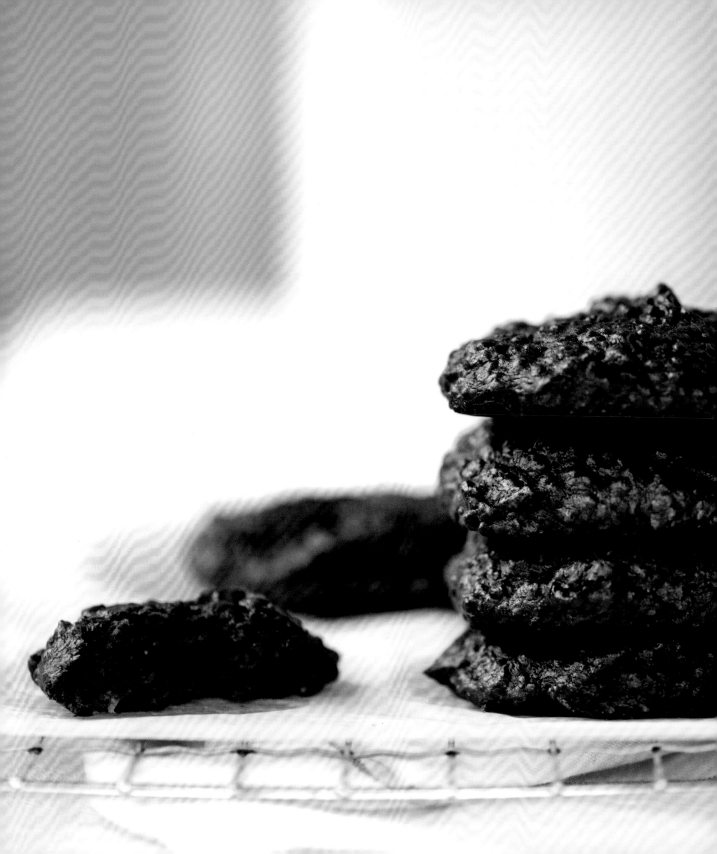

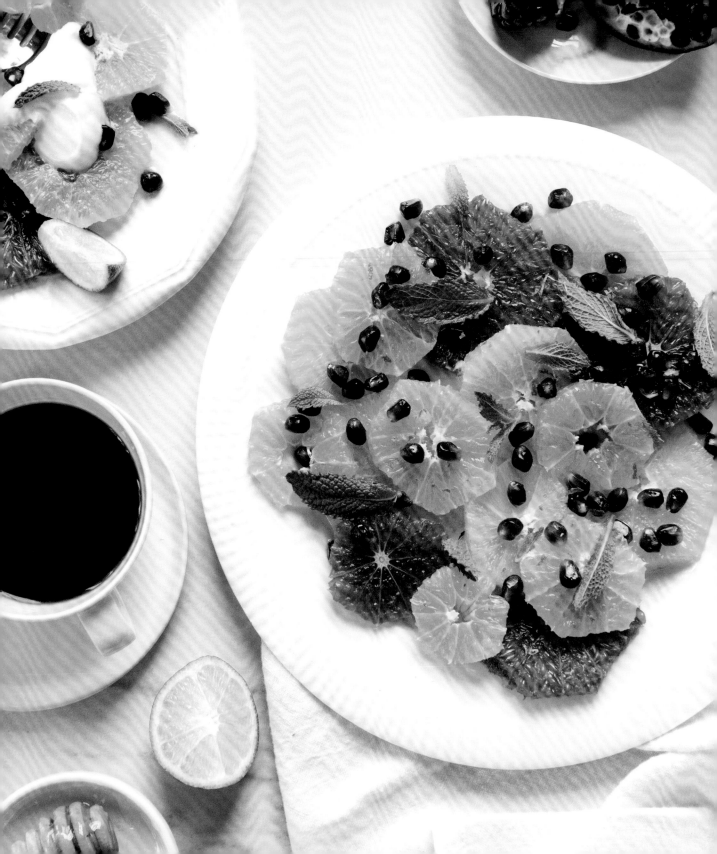

FRESH CITRUS SALAD

VEGETARIAN
VEGAN
DAIRY-FREE
WHEAT-FREE
PESCATARIAN

Citrus fruit is sweet, tart, and refreshing, especially at the peak of its season. When I've got an abundance of it, I always make this incredible Fresh Citrus Salad studded with lovely pomegranate and fresh mint. It's one of those dishes that looks really impressive but is actually effortless to make. It's almost too pretty to eat. Almost. I love it with a little coconut yogurt, but it can just as easily be enjoyed all on its own.

SERVINGS: **4**   PREP TIME: **15 MINUTES**

---

1 large grapefruit

2 navel oranges

4 mandarin oranges

¼ cup pomegranate seeds

2 teaspoons fresh mint

USING a sharp knife, carefully slice off the top and bottom of the grapefruit. Remove the peel by running the knife down along the sides of the grapefruit. Once the peel has been removed, turn the grapefruit on its side and slice it into ½-inch slices. Repeat with the remaining citrus fruits.

ARRANGE the citrus slices on a serving dish. Top with the pomegranate seeds and fresh mint.

ENJOY immediately or store in the refrigerator for up to 3 days.

simple swaps

Instead of fresh mint, try 2 teaspoons chopped fresh basil.

OVERNIGHT OATMEAL

VEGETARIAN
WHEAT-FREE
PESCATARIAN

Overnight oatmeal is truly a "meal made easy." You simply combine all the ingredients in a jar before bed, give them a shake, and then refrigerate them overnight. Come morning, you've got a filling, fiber-rich breakfast that is the definition of grab-and-go. Overnight oatmeal can be enjoyed hot or cold, and the flavor combinations are limited only by your imagination. I've included the classic recipe as well as three tasty twists you'll love.

CLASSIC OVERNIGHT OATMEAL

SERVINGS: **1**   PREP TIME: **3 MINUTES**

⅓ cup old-fashioned rolled oats

1 tablespoon chia seeds

⅓ cup 2% milk

2 teaspoons honey

IN a small container or mason jar, combine all the ingredients. Mix well, cover, and store in the refrigerator overnight. Come morning, enjoy the oatmeal cold, straight from the refrigerator, or heated in the microwave for 1 minute.

simple swaps

- You can use any type of milk in this recipe. I've tried it with dairy, almond, and soy milk. It's always delicious.
- Instead of honey, feel free to swap in some agave or maple syrup. Each of these sweeteners has a slightly different flavor, but they'll all be tasty.

mix it up

CHOCOLATE STRAWBERRY
½ teaspoon cocoa powder
¼ cup diced strawberries

BLUEBERRY LEMON
¼ cup fresh blueberries
¼ teaspoon grated lemon zest

POMEGRANATE PISTACHIO
¼ cup pomegranate seeds
1 tablespoon chopped shelled pistachios

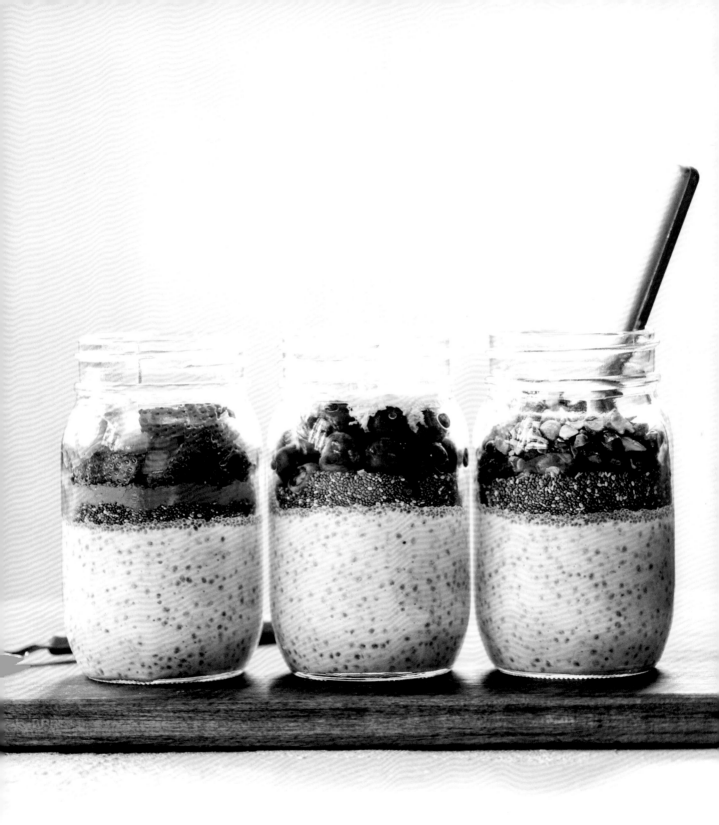

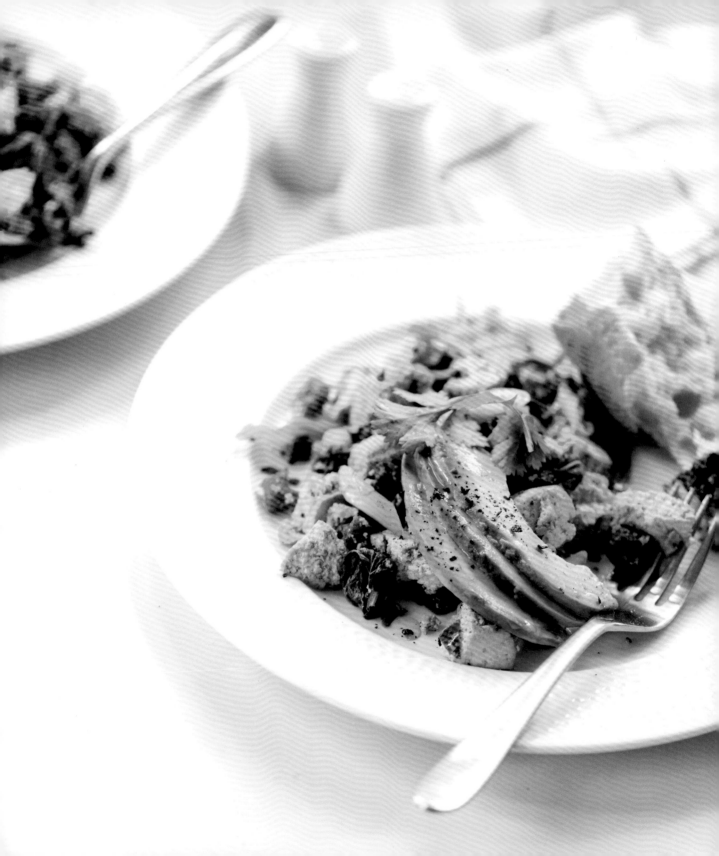

VEGAN TOFU SCRAMBLE

This vegan tofu scramble is a great way to get your plant-based protein in first thing. Unlike traditional scrambled eggs, this dish can be prepared in advance and reheated when you're ready to enjoy it, so it's a great make-ahead option to include in your Sunday meal prep.

VEGETARIAN
VEGAN
DAIRY-FREE
PESCATARIAN

SERVINGS: **2**   PREP TIME: **10 MINUTES**   COOK TIME: **8 MINUTES**

1 tablespoon coconut oil

1 red bell pepper, finely diced

8 ounces extra-firm tofu, crumbled

1 tablespoon soy sauce

½ teaspoon ground turmeric

½ teaspoon garlic powder

¼ teaspoon red pepper flakes

2 cups chopped baby spinach (3 to 4 ounces)

3 green onions, finely sliced

Salt and freshly ground black pepper

Avocado slices, for serving

Fresh cilantro, for serving

IN a large skillet, melt the coconut oil over medium-high heat. Add the bell pepper and cook, stirring often, until it softens, about 4 minutes. Add the tofu, soy sauce, turmeric, garlic powder, and red pepper flakes and cook, stirring often, until the tofu is heated through, about 2 minutes. Add the spinach and green onions and cook, stirring, until the spinach is completely wilted, 2 minutes. Season with salt and pepper.

SERVE immediately with sliced avocado and fresh cilantro, or let cool completely and store in the refrigerator for up to 3 days.

mix it up

If you want to amp up the veggie factor even more in this dish, consider adding 1 cup broccoli florets, 1 cup halved snap peas, or 1 cup finely chopped kale leaves with the bell pepper at the start of cooking.

CHEWY GRANOLA BARS

VEGETARIAN
WHEAT-FREE
DAIRY-FREE
PESCATARIAN

If I'm being honest, it took me months to perfect this recipe. I went through so many variations, but the results were either too crumbly, too firm, too sweet, or too difficult to make. I kind of felt like Goldilocks when I finally got them just right. These granola bars are soft and chewy and just sweet enough to satisfy. As a bonus, the classic recipe is nut-free so they're perfect for school lunches.

SERVINGS: **8**   PREP TIME: **25 MINUTES**   COOK TIME: **5 TO 7 MINUTES**

1½ cups old-fashioned rolled oats

½ cup raw pumpkin seeds

½ cup raw sunflower seeds

Cooking spray

1 cup pitted dates

½ cup dried cranberries

¼ cup honey

½ teaspoon sea salt

PREHEAT the oven to 350°F.

SPREAD the oats, pumpkin seeds, and sunflower seeds in a single layer on a baking sheet. Bake for 5 to 7 minutes, until they are lightly toasted.

IN the meantime, grease an 8 x 8-inch baking dish with cooking spray and then line it with parchment paper, leaving an overhang to make the granola easy to remove.

IN a food processor, pulse the dates until they are smooth and a sticky ball forms.

TRANSFER the dates to a large bowl. Add the toasted oats and seeds, dried cranberries, honey, and salt. Use your hands to mix the ingredients until they are very well combined. (To prevent the mixture from sticking to your hands, grease them with a little coconut oil or butter.)

TRANSFER the mixture to the prepared baking dish and press it firmly to form a dense, even layer. Freeze for 15 minutes.

USING the overhanging parchment paper, gently transfer the granola to a cutting board. Use a sharp knife to cut it into bars or squares.

STORE in the refrigerator for up to 1 week or in the freezer for up to 3 months. I recommend wrapping each granola bar or square individually in parchment paper to prevent them from sticking together and to help make them easier to grab on the go.

(continued)

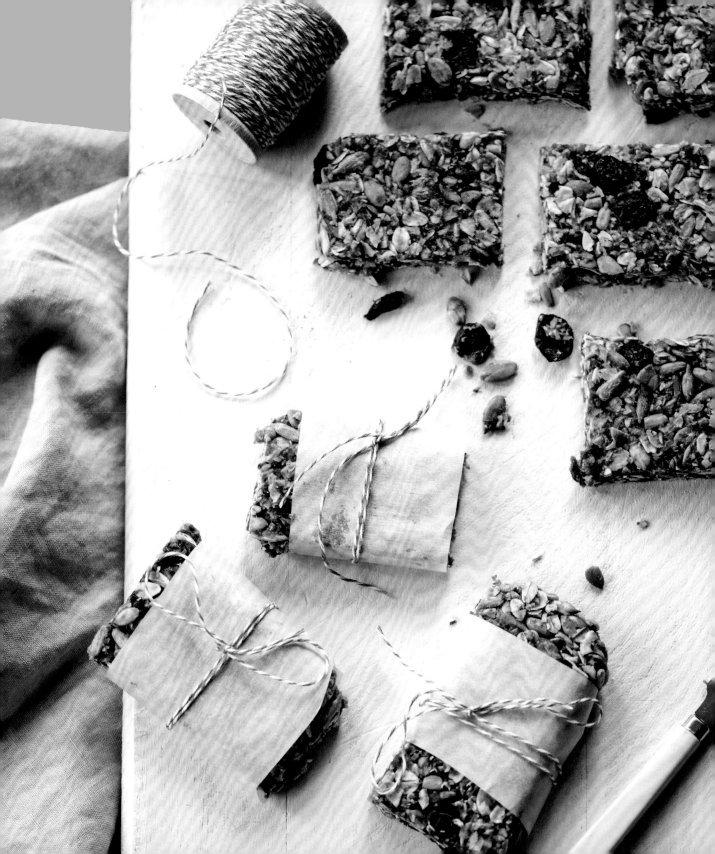

(Chewy Granola Bars continued)

mix it up

CHERRY-ALMOND GRANOLA BARS
Replace the pumpkin seeds with ½ cup chopped raw almonds. Instead of dried cranberries, use ½ cup dried cherries.

APPLE-CINNAMON GRANOLA BARS
Use ½ cup chopped dried apple in place of the dried cranberries. Omit the sea salt and add 1 teaspoon ground cinnamon.

CHOCOLATE-HAZELNUT GRANOLA BARS
Replace the pumpkin and sunflower seeds with 1 cup chopped raw hazelnuts. Just before pulsing the dates in the food processor, add 2 teaspoons unsweetened cocoa powder. Instead of dried cranberries, add ½ cup semisweet chocolate chips.

simple swaps

- You can swap the seeds in this recipe for chopped peanuts, almonds, hazelnuts, pistachios, or walnuts. It's important to use raw nuts because you'll be toasting them in the oven, and nuts that are already toasted may burn.
- The dried cranberries can easily be replaced by almost any dried fruit—raisins, dried apricots, dried mango, and dried blueberries all make delicious choices.

HEALTHY BREAKFAST WRAPS

Breakfast wraps are a great way to eat on the go. Unlike traditional breakfast wraps that include things like bacon and eggs, these versions don't require any cooking, so you or your kids can put them together quickly and get out the door on busy mornings. Plus, they're bursting with ingredients you can feel really good about.

PB&J BREAKFAST WRAP

VEGETARIAN
DAIRY-FREE
PESCATARIAN

SERVINGS: **1**   PREP TIME: **5 MINUTES**

2 tablespoons smooth natural peanut butter

1 tablespoon strawberry jam

1 large whole wheat tortilla

⅓ cup sliced strawberries

¼ cup granola

2 tablespoons chopped peanuts

SPREAD the peanut butter and jam on the tortilla. Top with the strawberries, granola, and peanuts. Roll up the tortilla and enjoy immediately.

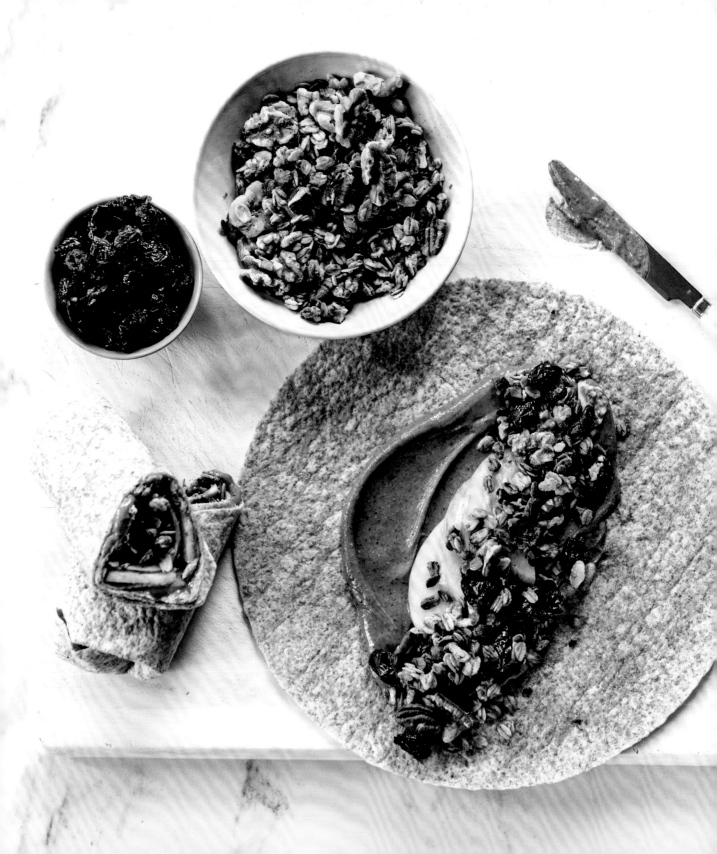

BLUEBERRY COCONUT BREAKFAST WRAP

VEGETARIAN

PESCATARIAN

SERVINGS: **1**   PREP TIME: **5 MINUTES**

2 tablespoons coconut-
  flavored Greek yogurt

1 large whole wheat tortilla

⅓ cup blueberries

¼ cup granola

2 tablespoons coconut chips

SPREAD the yogurt on the tortilla. Top with the blueberries, granola, and coconut chips. Roll up the tortilla and enjoy immediately.

CRUNCHY APPLE & ALMOND BUTTER BREAKFAST WRAP

VEGETARIAN

DAIRY-FREE

PESCATARIAN

SERVINGS: **1**   PREP TIME: **5 MINUTES**

2 tablespoons smooth natural
  almond butter

1 large whole wheat tortilla

1 apple, cored and thinly
  sliced

¼ cup granola

2 tablespoons dried
  cranberries

SPREAD the almond butter on the tortilla. Top with the apple, granola, and dried cranberries. Roll up the tortilla and enjoy immediately.

GOOD MORNING MUFFINS

VEGETARIAN
PESCATARIAN

I call these Good Morning Muffins because they are just bursting with good-for-you ingredients like carrot, apple, and pecans, making them a great way to start your day. They're also loaded with protein and fiber to help keep you full longer. Plus, they taste as good as they look thanks to an abundance of delicious spice.

SERVINGS: 12   PREP TIME: **10 MINUTES**   COOK TIME: **25 TO 30 MINUTES**

Cooking spray (optional)

1½ cups whole wheat flour

1 cup old-fashioned rolled oats

¾ cup coconut sugar

2 tablespoons ground flaxseed

1 tablespoon baking powder

2 teaspoons ground cinnamon

1 teaspoon ground ginger

1 cup plain Greek yogurt

½ cup 2% milk

2 large eggs

1 cup shredded carrots (about 2 medium)

1 cup shredded apples (about 2 small)

¼ cup dried cranberries

¼ cup chopped pecans

PREHEAT the oven to 350°F. Grease a 12-cup muffin pan lightly with cooking spray or use silicone baking cups.

IN a large bowl, whisk together the flour, oats, coconut sugar, flaxseed, baking powder, cinnamon, and ginger until thoroughly combined. Add the yogurt, milk, and eggs and stir well. Fold in the carrots, apples, cranberries, and pecans.

SCOOP the batter into the prepared muffin pan. Bake for 25 to 30 minutes, until just golden on top. Remove the muffins from the pan and let cool for at least 5 minutes.

SERVE warm from the oven or at room temperature, or store in the refrigerator for up to 5 days or in the freezer for up to 3 months.

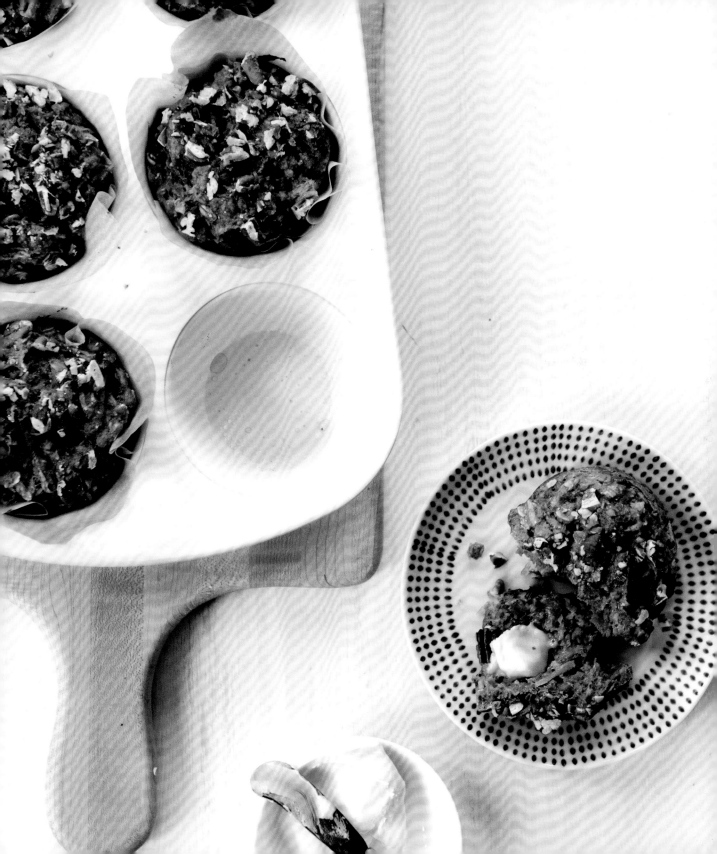

EASY BAKED EGGS

These delicious Easy Baked Egg ideas are perfect for weekend brunch. They're simple enough to pull together quickly, but fancy enough to serve to guests. I especially love the fact that they're made in individual servings so they're completely customizable based on someone's tastes. I like to serve them with my Crispy Smashed Potatoes (page 60) and toast for dipping.

MUSHROOM & GOAT CHEESE BAKED EGGS

SERVINGS: **2**   PREP TIME: **5 MINUTES**   COOK TIME: **10 TO 12 MINUTES**

VEGETARIAN
WHEAT-FREE
PESCATARIAN

1 teaspoon vegetable oil

½ cup thinly sliced cremini mushrooms

¼ cup crumbled goat cheese

4 large eggs

Salt and freshly ground black pepper

½ teaspoon fresh thyme leaves

PREHEAT the oven to 425°F. Lightly grease two ramekins or small oven-safe dishes with the vegetable oil.

DIVIDE the mushrooms and goat cheese evenly between the ramekins. Create a small well in the center of the ingredients. Crack 2 eggs into each well. Season with salt and pepper and top with the thyme leaves.

BAKE for 10 to 12 minutes, until the egg whites are set and the yolks are cooked to your liking.

SERVE immediately.

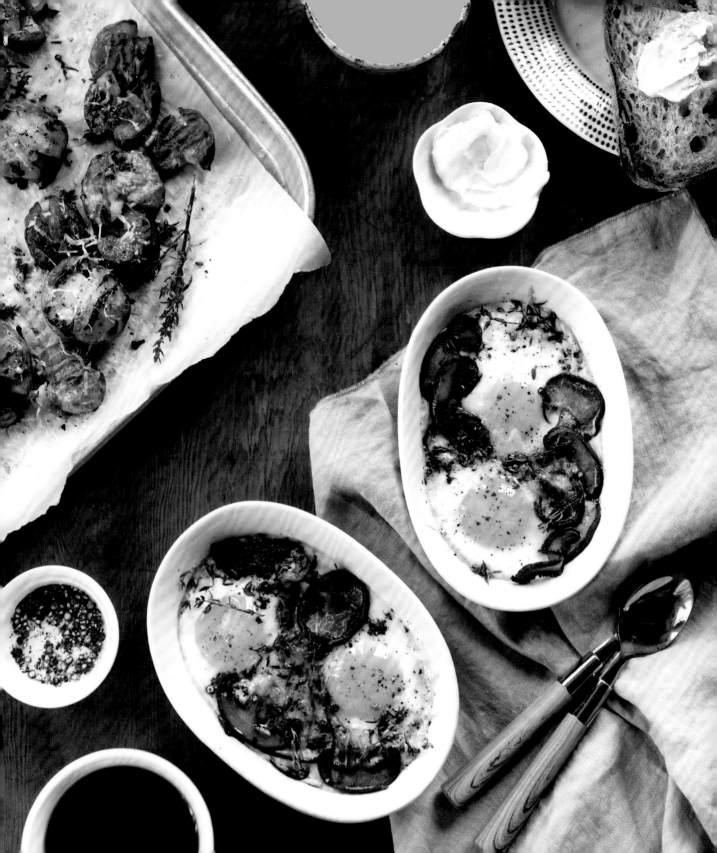

CAPRESE BAKED EGGS

SERVINGS: **2**   PREP TIME: **5 MINUTES**   COOK TIME: **10 TO 12 MINUTES**

VEGETARIAN
WHEAT-FREE
PESCATARIAN

1 teaspoon vegetable oil

⅔ cup halved cherry tomatoes

¼ cup grated mozzarella cheese

4 large eggs

¼ teaspoon red pepper flakes (optional)

Salt and freshly ground black pepper

1 tablespoon finely chopped fresh basil

PREHEAT the oven to 425°F. Lightly grease two ramekins or small oven-safe dishes with the vegetable oil.

DIVIDE the tomatoes and mozzarella evenly between the ramekins. Create a small well in the center of the ingredients. Crack 2 eggs into each well. Season with red pepper flakes (if using), and salt and pepper.

BAKE for 10 to 12 minutes, until the egg whites are set and the yolks are cooked to your liking.

TOP with the fresh basil and serve immediately.

HAM, SWISS & ASPARAGUS BAKED EGGS

WHEAT-FREE

SERVINGS: **2**   PREP TIME: **5 MINUTES**   COOK TIME: **10 TO 12 MINUTES**

1 teaspoon vegetable oil

½ cup chopped asparagus

½ cup chopped deli ham

¼ cup grated Swiss cheese

4 large eggs

Salt and freshly ground black pepper

PREHEAT the oven to 425°F. Lightly grease two ramekins or small oven-safe dishes with the vegetable oil.

DIVIDE the asparagus, ham, and Swiss cheese evenly between the ramekins. Create a small well in the center of the ingredients. Crack 2 eggs into each well. Season with salt and pepper.

BAKE for 10 to 12 minutes, until the egg whites are set and the yolks are cooked to your liking.

SERVE immediately.

CRISPY SMASHED POTATOES

Crispy Smashed Potatoes just make brunch better. They're flavorful and filling and always worth the extra effort. When I serve them to guests, there are never any leftovers, which to me is a surefire sign of success. I hope you love them as much as I do!

SERVINGS: **4**   PREP TIME: **5 MINUTES**   COOK TIME: **40 MINUTES**

---

24 baby potatoes

1 tablespoon extra-virgin olive oil

1 teaspoon garlic powder

1 teaspoon paprika

2 teaspoons fresh thyme leaves

Salt and freshly ground black pepper

3 tablespoons freshly grated Parmesan cheese

PREHEAT the oven to 425°F.

PUT the potatoes in a large pot and add water to cover. Bring the water to a boil and cook the potatoes until they are fork-tender, 10 to 12 minutes. Drain and rinse under cold water until they are cool enough to handle.

ON a baking sheet, smash each potato with the palm of your hand or the bottom of a small bowl or glass. Brush each potato with the olive oil and season them liberally with the garlic powder, paprika, thyme, and salt and pepper.

BAKE for 20 to 25 minutes, until golden. Remove the potatoes from the oven and switch the oven to the broil setting.

TOP the potatoes evenly with the Parmesan and broil for about 3 minutes, until they become crisp on top.

SERVE immediately.

mix it up

With these tasty taters, the seasoning possibilities are virtually endless. You can swap the seasonings in the classic recipe for 2 tablespoons Greek Seasoning (page 230), Ranch Seasoning (page 231), or Cajun Seasoning (page 231) instead.

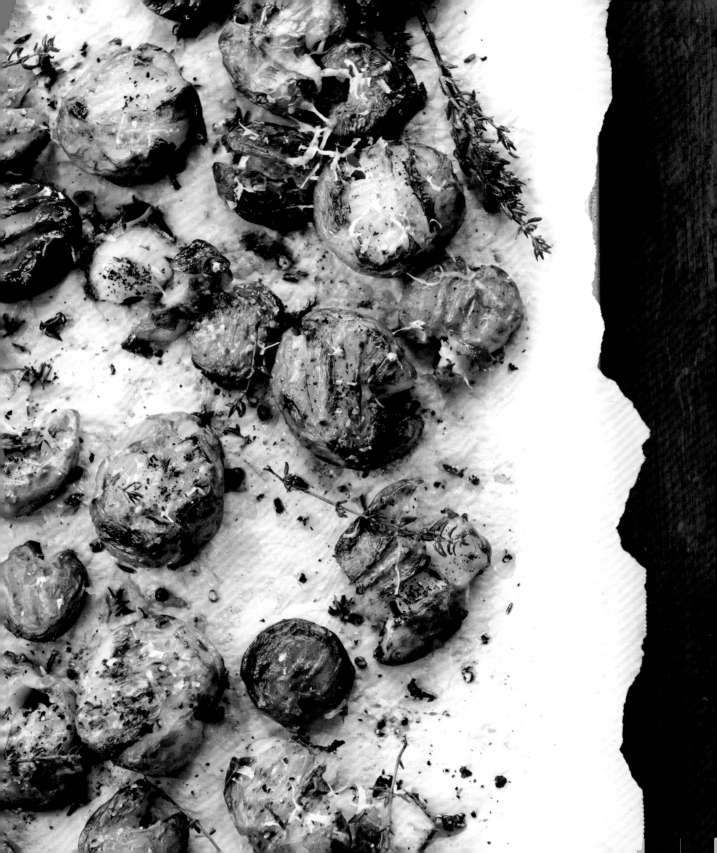

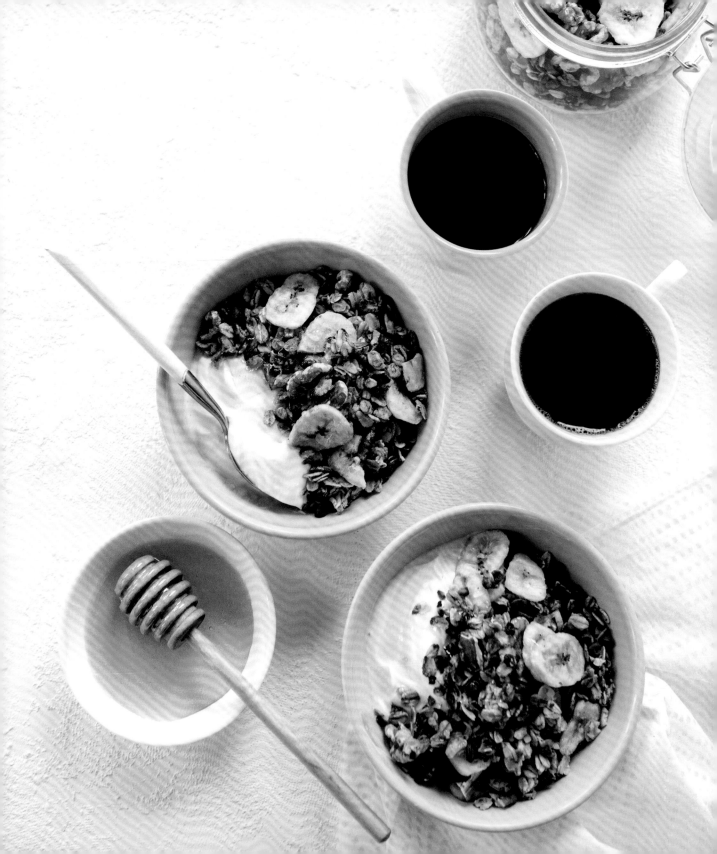

HOMEMADE GRANOLA

Granola is so easy to make, it's a wonder to me that anyone bothers to buy it anymore. When you make your granola from scratch, you can control the amount of added sugar and avoid any unnecessary preservatives. Plus, with all the flavor possibilities, you're sure to please even the pickiest eaters at home. Here are three of my favorites . . .

BANANA BREAD GRANOLA

VEGETARIAN
WHEAT-FREE
PESCATARIAN

SERVINGS: **8**   PREP TIME: **5 MINUTES**   COOK TIME: **20 MINUTES**

1 large ripe banana, mashed

⅓ cup maple syrup

¼ cup coconut oil, melted

1 teaspoon vanilla extract

1 teaspoon ground cinnamon

3 cups old-fashioned rolled oats

½ cup chopped raw pecans

½ cup chopped raw walnuts

¼ cup vegan dark chocolate chips

½ cup banana chips

Vanilla yogurt, for serving

Honey, for serving

PREHEAT the oven to 350°F. Line a baking sheet with parchment paper.

IN a large bowl, combine the mashed banana, maple syrup, coconut oil, vanilla, and cinnamon. Mix well. Add the oats, pecans, and walnuts and stir until everything is well combined.

POUR the mixture onto the prepared baking sheet and spread it into an even layer. Sprinkle with the chocolate chips and bake for about 20 minutes, until the granola is crisp and golden.

REMOVE the granola from the oven and let cool completely. Stir in the banana chips.

SERVE immediately with some vanilla yogurt and a drizzle of honey, or transfer to an airtight container and store at room temperature or in the refrigerator for up to 1 week.

VERY BERRY ALMOND GRANOLA

SERVINGS: **8**   PREP TIME: **5 MINUTES**   COOK TIME: **25 MINUTES**

¾ cup smooth natural almond butter

⅓ cup maple syrup

¼ cup coconut oil

3 cups old-fashioned rolled oats

¾ cup chopped raw almonds

½ cup mixed dried berries (I like dried strawberries, blueberries, and cherries)

PREHEAT the oven to 350°F. Line a baking sheet with parchment paper.

IN a large saucepan, combine the almond butter, maple syrup, and coconut oil. Heat over medium heat, stirring continuously, until the mixture is smooth, 3 to 4 minutes. Add the oats and almonds and stir until well combined.

POUR the mixture onto the prepared baking sheet and spread it into an even layer. Bake for about 20 minutes, until the granola is crisp and golden.

REMOVE the granola from the oven and let cool completely. Stir in the dried berries.

SERVE immediately or transfer to an airtight container and store at room temperature or in the refrigerator for up to 1 week.

SAVORY SPICED GRANOLA

VEGETARIAN
DAIRY-FREE
WHEAT-FREE
PESCATARIAN

SERVINGS: **8**   PREP TIME: **5 MINUTES**   COOK TIME: **20 MINUTES**

1 egg white

¼ cup extra-virgin olive oil

2 tablespoons honey

2 teaspoons chopped fresh rosemary

1 teaspoon garlic powder

1 teaspoon smoked paprika

¼ teaspoon cayenne pepper (optional)

3 cups old-fashioned rolled oats

½ cup chopped raw almonds

½ cup chopped raw walnuts

¼ cup raw sunflower seeds

Salt and freshly ground black pepper

PREHEAT the oven to 350°F. Line a baking sheet with parchment paper.

IN a large bowl, whisk the egg white until frothy. Add the olive oil, honey, rosemary, garlic powder, paprika, and cayenne (if using). Mix well. Add the oats, almonds, walnuts, and sunflower seeds and stir until well combined.

POUR the mixture onto the prepared baking sheet and spread it into an even layer. Season liberally with salt and black pepper. Bake for about 20 minutes, until the granola is crisp and golden.

REMOVE the granola from the oven and let cool completely.

SERVE immediately or transfer to an airtight container and store at room temperature or in the refrigerator for up to 1 week.

SAVORY HAM & SWISS STRATA

This Savory Ham & Swiss Strata is an ideal brunch dish to serve a crowd. The best part is that it can be prepared the night before and then baked just before serving, so it's perfect for entertaining. If you've never had strata before, it's basically like a rich, savory bread pudding that's guaranteed to satisfy.

SERVINGS: **6**   PREP TIME: **1 HOUR 15 MINUTES**   COOK TIME: **55 MINUTES**

---

1 tablespoon butter

1 loaf crusty French bread, cut into ½-inch cubes

8 slices deli ham, chopped

3 green onions, finely chopped

1 cup grated Gruyère cheese

8 large eggs

½ cup 2% milk

½ cup heavy cream

Salt and freshly ground black pepper

GREASE a large baking dish with the butter.

LAYER in half the bread, ham, green onions, and Gruyère. Add a second layer of bread, ham, and green onions. Reserve the remaining cheese.

IN a large bowl, whisk together the eggs, milk, cream, and salt and pepper. Pour the egg mixture evenly over the ingredients in the baking dish. Top evenly with the remaining Gruyère. Cover the dish with aluminum foil and refrigerate for at least 1 hour or ideally overnight.

WHEN ready to bake the strata, preheat the oven to 350°F.

BAKE the strata for 40 minutes with the foil on. Remove the foil and bake for 15 minutes more, or until the top is crisp and golden.

SERVE immediately.

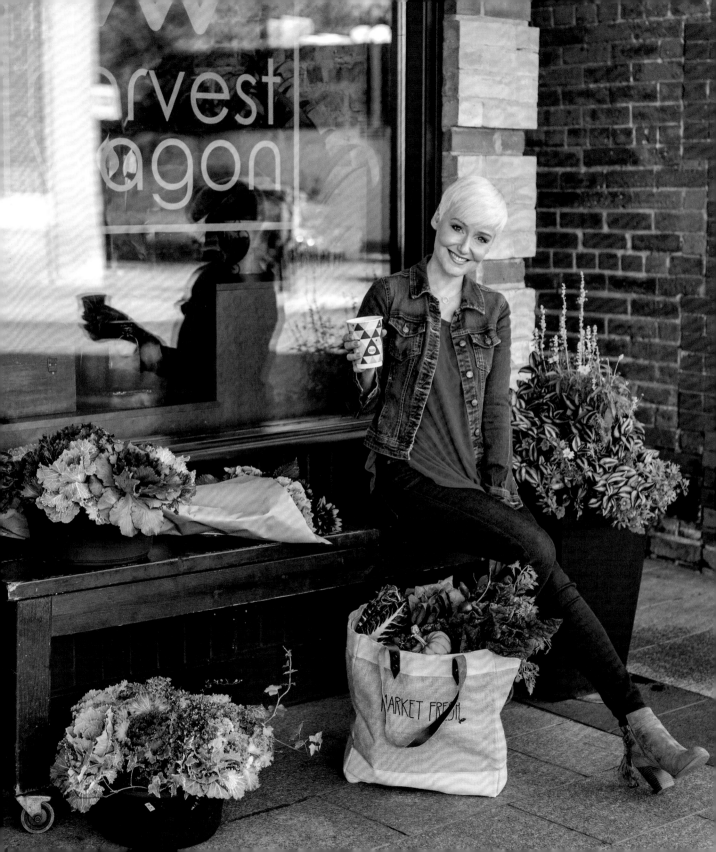

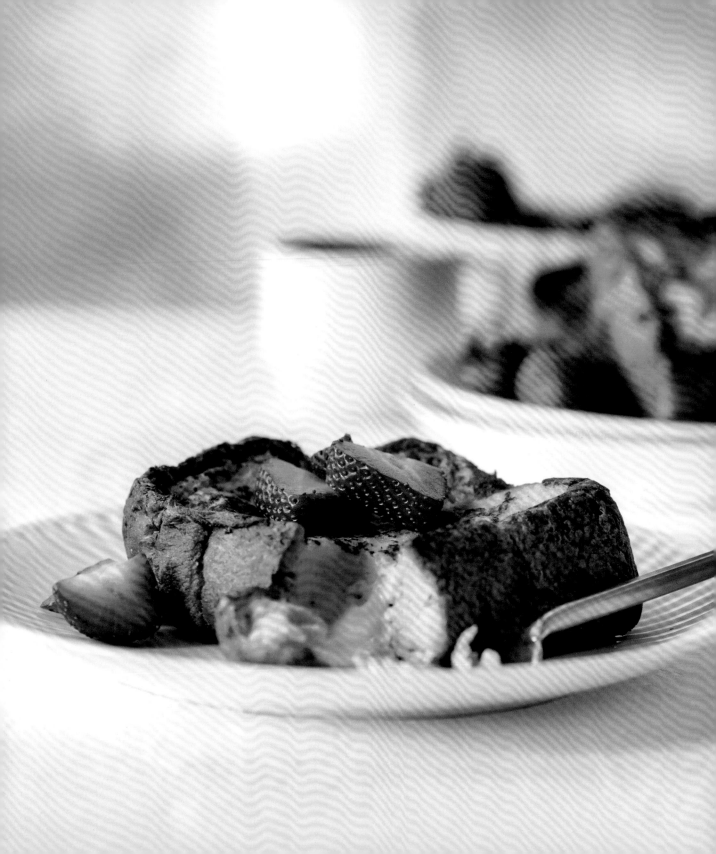

STRAWBERRY-STUFFED FRENCH TOAST

This showstopping recipe is totally brunch-worthy and easier to make than you might think. And of course, the fact that it tastes like strawberry cheesecake means it's pretty much guaranteed to please a crowd.

SERVINGS: **4**   PREP TIME: **10 MINUTES**   COOK TIME: **30 MINUTES**

---

6 ounces cream cheese, at room temperature

½ cup diced strawberries

Grated zest and juice of ½ lemon

1 crusty French loaf

3 large eggs

⅓ cup 2% milk

1 teaspoon vanilla extract

2 tablespoons butter

½ cup maple syrup, for serving

IN the bowl of a stand mixer fitted with the paddle attachment or in a large bowl using a hand mixer, beat the cream cheese, strawberries, lemon zest, and lemon juice until smooth.

USING a sharp serrated knife, cut four 1½-inch-thick slices of bread. Using a small serrated knife, cut a pocket into the top of each slice of bread, being sure not to cut all the way through. Fill each pocket with the strawberry–cream cheese mixture.

IN a shallow bowl, whisk together eggs, milk, and vanilla.

IN a nonstick skillet, melt ½ tablespoon of the butter over medium heat. Dip a slice of bread into the egg mixture, coating it on both sides, then transfer it to the pan. Fry until golden on one side, about 3 minutes, then flip it with a spatula and fry on the second side for 2 minutes. Transfer to a plate and repeat to cook the remaining French toast.

SERVE immediately, with maple syrup.

mix it up

While Strawberry-Stuffed French Toast is a classic, you can always swap out the strawberries in the filling for ½ cup blueberries, 1 chopped large banana, or even ½ cup chocolate chips. Yum!

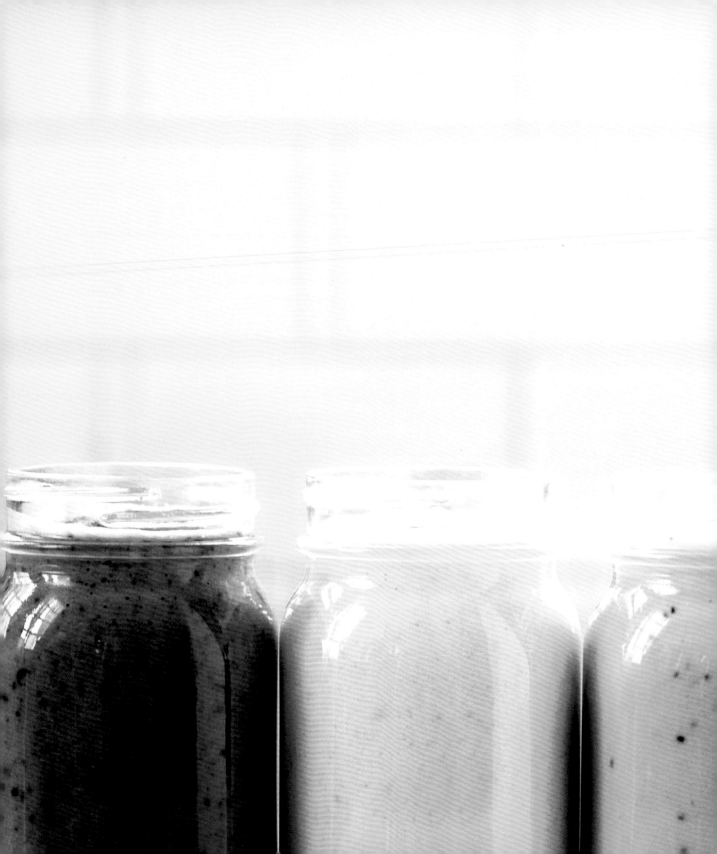

5 HEALTHY BREAKFAST SMOOTHIES

As far as I'm concerned, smoothies are the best way to start your day. They're loaded with nutrients, effortless to prepare, and perfect on the go. Not to mention the fact that the flavor possibilities are simply endless. Here are a few of my very favorites . . .

CREAMY ORANGE SMOOTHIE

VEGETARIAN
WHEAT-FREE
PESCATARIAN

SERVINGS: **1**   PREP TIME: **5 MINUTES**

¾ cup orange juice

1 large ripe banana

½ cup vanilla Greek yogurt

1 small orange, peeled

½ peach, pitted

½ teaspoon ground turmeric

COMBINE all the ingredients in a blender and blend until smooth. Enjoy immediately.

VEGETARIAN
WHEAT-FREE
PESCATARIAN

PB&J SMOOTHIE

SERVINGS: **1**   PREP TIME: **5 MINUTES**

¾ cup unsweetened almond milk

½ cup vanilla Greek yogurt

1 large ripe banana

4 strawberries, hulled

1 tablespoon smooth natural peanut butter

COMBINE all the ingredients in a blender and blend until smooth. Enjoy immediately.

TROPICAL SUNSHINE SMOOTHIE

VEGETARIAN

VEGAN

DAIRY-FREE

WHEAT-FREE

PESCATARIAN

SERVINGS: **1**   PREP TIME: **5 MINUTES**

¾ cup unsweetened almond milk

1 large ripe banana

½ cup diced pineapple

½ cup diced mango

½ teaspoon grated fresh ginger

COMBINE all the ingredients in a blender and blend until smooth. Enjoy immediately.

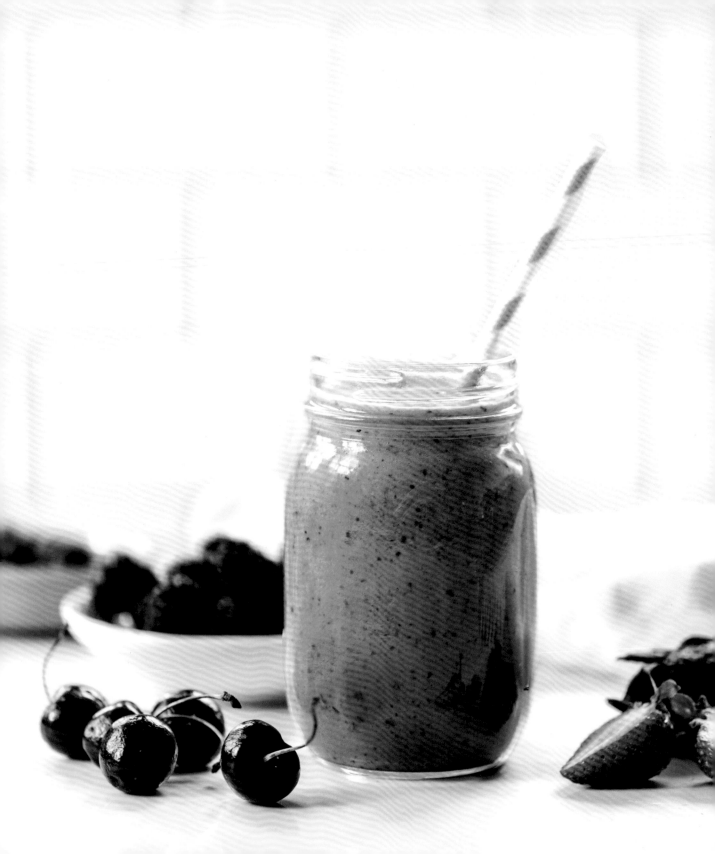

VANILLA BERRY BLISS SMOOTHIE

SERVINGS: **1**   PREP TIME: **5 MINUTES**

¾ cup unsweetened almond milk

1 large ripe banana

½ cup quartered strawberries

½ cup blueberries

½ cup blackberries

½ cup frozen pitted cherries (they're more affordable than fresh)

2 tablespoons vanilla protein powder

COMBINE all the ingredients in a blender and blend until smooth. Enjoy immediately.

GO GREEN SMOOTHIE

SERVINGS: **1** PREP TIME: **5 MINUTES**

¾ cup orange juice

1 large ripe banana

½ cup vanilla Greek yogurt

1 cup baby spinach (1½ to 2 ounces)

2 kiwis, peeled

½ avocado

COMBINE all the ingredients in a blender and blend until smooth. Enjoy immediately.

smoothie tips

1. Add the liquid first, so it's close to the blades, for easier blending.

2. Use frozen fruit instead of adding ice so you don't water down your smoothie.

3. Sweeten things up by adding a touch of honey, agave syrup, maple syrup, or pitted dates. Soak dates in water for 5 to 10 minutes, then drain, to make them softer and easier to blend.

4. Make your smoothie even more nutritious by adding 1 tablespoon hemp, flax, or chia seeds. You can also add ¼ cup old-fashioned oats or cooked quinoa for protein and fiber.

5. To make your mornings even easier, prepackage your smoothie ingredients (except for the liquids) in individual zipper bags and keep them in the freezer. Then simply put your liquids in the blender, pour in the contents of the bag, and blend until smooth.

simple swaps

- Almond milk can be swapped out for dairy, hemp, soy, or oat milk based on your preferences.
- For those of you who aren't big fans of bananas, you can always replace the banana with ½ cup vanilla Greek yogurt. You'll get a similar creamy texture and that same touch of sweetness the banana provides.

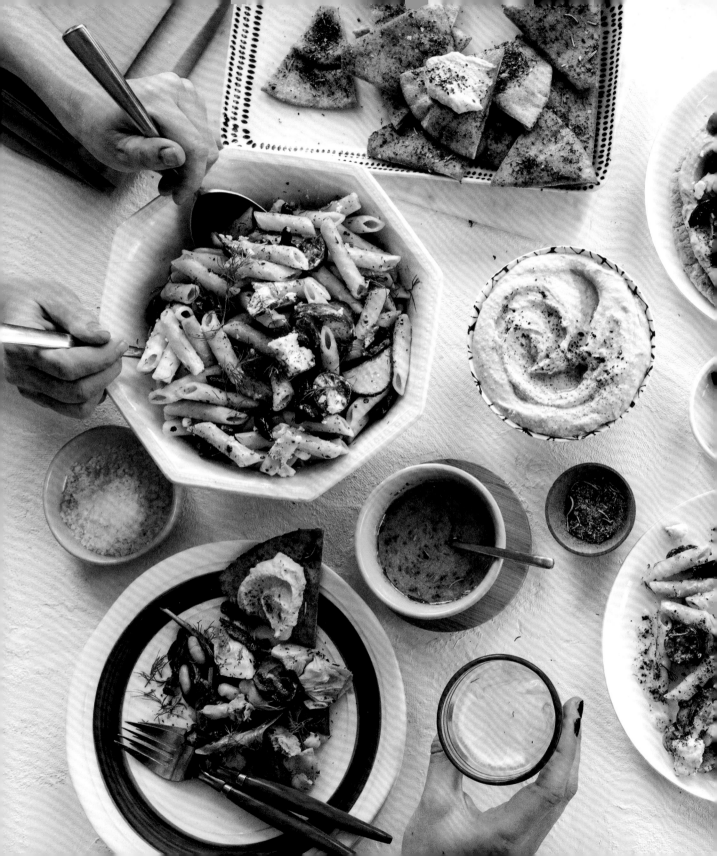

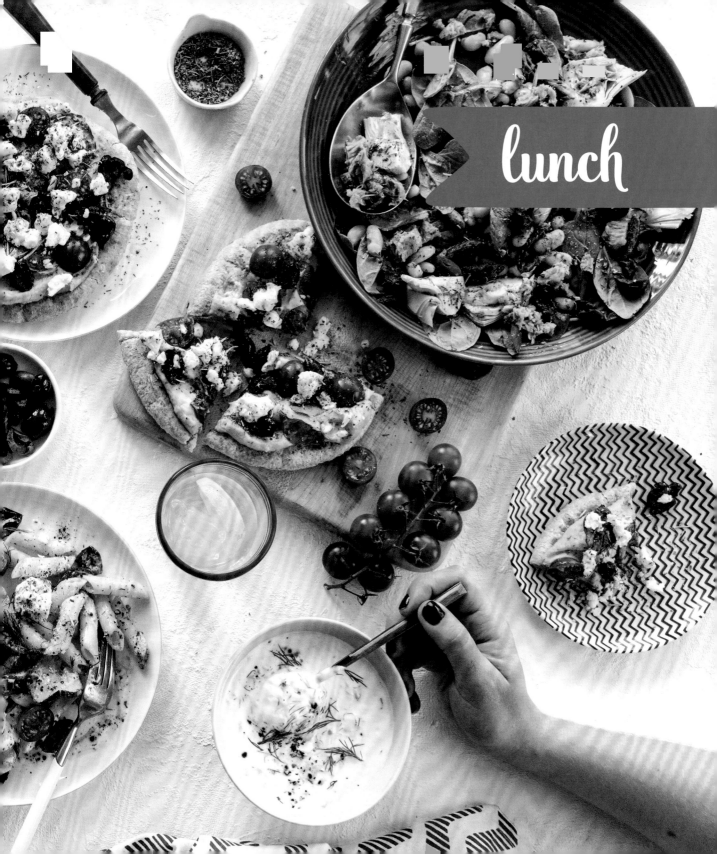

lunch

TANGY THAI QUINOA

VEGETARIAN

DAIRY-FREE

PESCATARIAN

This satisfying salad boasts a bounty of delicious Asian-inspired flavors. It's chock-full of rainbow-colored veggies like bell pepper, cabbage, and carrot so you know it's as nutritious as it is delicious. Plus, the addition of quinoa boosts the protein factor so you're sure to feel fuller longer.

SERVINGS: **2**   PREP TIME: **10 MINUTES**

2 tablespoons soy sauce

1 tablespoon smooth natural peanut butter

1 teaspoon honey

Juice of 1 lime

1 garlic clove, minced

½ teaspoon grated fresh ginger

¼ teaspoon red pepper flakes (optional)

3 cups cooked quinoa (see page 34)

1 red bell pepper, diced

1 cup shredded red cabbage

2 medium carrots, shredded

½ cup frozen shelled edamame, cooked

IN a small bowl, whisk together the soy sauce, peanut butter, honey, lime juice, garlic, ginger, and red pepper flakes (if using) until well combined.

IN a large bowl, mix the quinoa, bell pepper, red cabbage, carrots, and edamame. Pour the dressing over the salad and toss until everything is evenly dressed.

SERVE immediately or store in the refrigerator for up to 4 days.

simple swaps

- The quinoa in this dish can easily be swapped out for cooked brown rice or rice noodles.
- To create a peanut-free version of this dish, use tahini in place of the peanut butter.

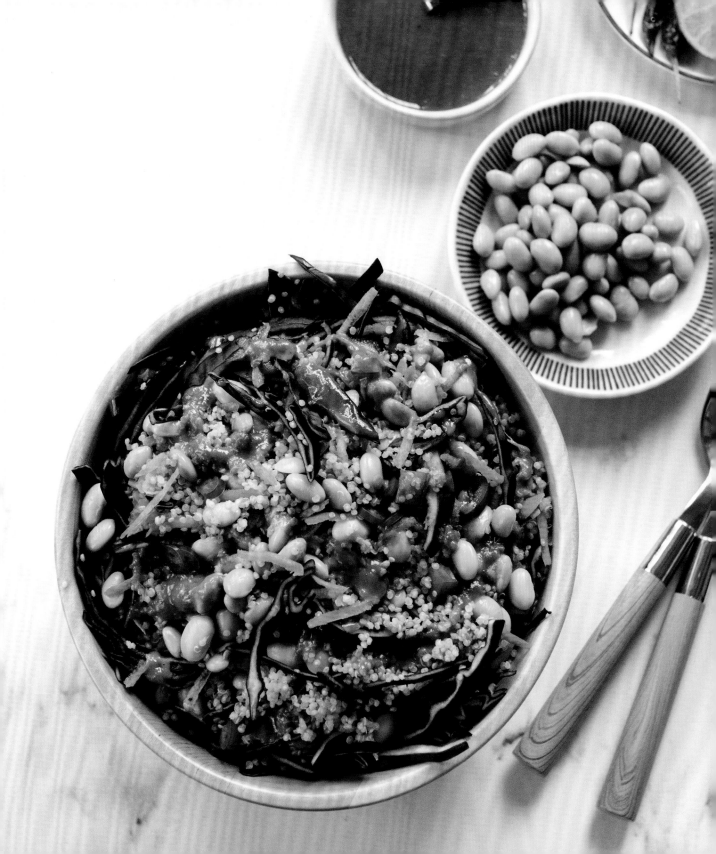

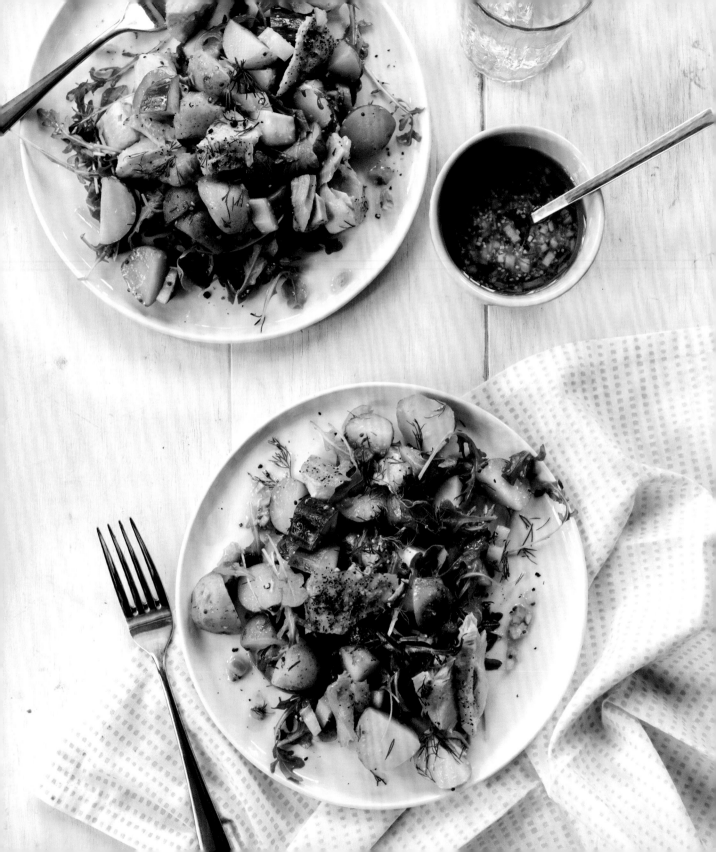

FRESH POTATO SALAD WITH SALMON

WHEAT-FREE
DAIRY-FREE
PESCATARIAN

The mention of potato salad usually conjures an image of a gloppy, mayo-laden mess, which is why I find Fresh Potato Salad tossed in a light but flavorful vinaigrette so much more appealing. This tasty take has lots of crunch courtesy of some crisp cucumber and celery and is surprisingly filling thanks to the addition of tender flaked salmon. It is by far my favorite spring dish.

SERVINGS: **2**   PREP TIME: **10 MINUTES**   COOK TIME: **15 MINUTES**

¼ cup extra-virgin olive oil

3 tablespoons red wine vinegar

1 tablespoon grainy Dijon mustard

1 shallot, minced

1 teaspoon prepared horseradish

Salt and freshly ground black pepper

1 (8-ounce) salmon fillet

1 pound new potatoes, quartered

½ English cucumber, diced

3 celery stalks, diced

2 tablespoons chopped fresh dill

6 cups arugula

PREHEAT the oven to 400°F. Line a baking sheet with parchment paper.

IN a small bowl, whisk together the olive oil, vinegar, mustard, shallot, horseradish, and salt and pepper.

ARRANGE the salmon fillet on the prepared baking sheet. Season liberally with salt and pepper. Bake for about 15 minutes, until the salmon is cooked through. Remove the salmon from the oven and flake it with a fork. Set aside to cool.

WHILE the salmon is cooking, use a large pot with a steamer insert to steam the potatoes until they're fork-tender, about 12 minutes. Transfer to a bowl lined with a paper towel and let cool completely.

IN a large bowl, combine the potatoes, cucumber, celery, and dill. Pour over the dressing and toss gently until everything is well coated.

ARRANGE the potato salad on a bed of arugula and top with the flaked salmon. Serve immediately or store in the refrigerator for up to 3 days.

mix it up

Try adding some thinly sliced radishes, steamed asparagus, or spring peas to the salad.

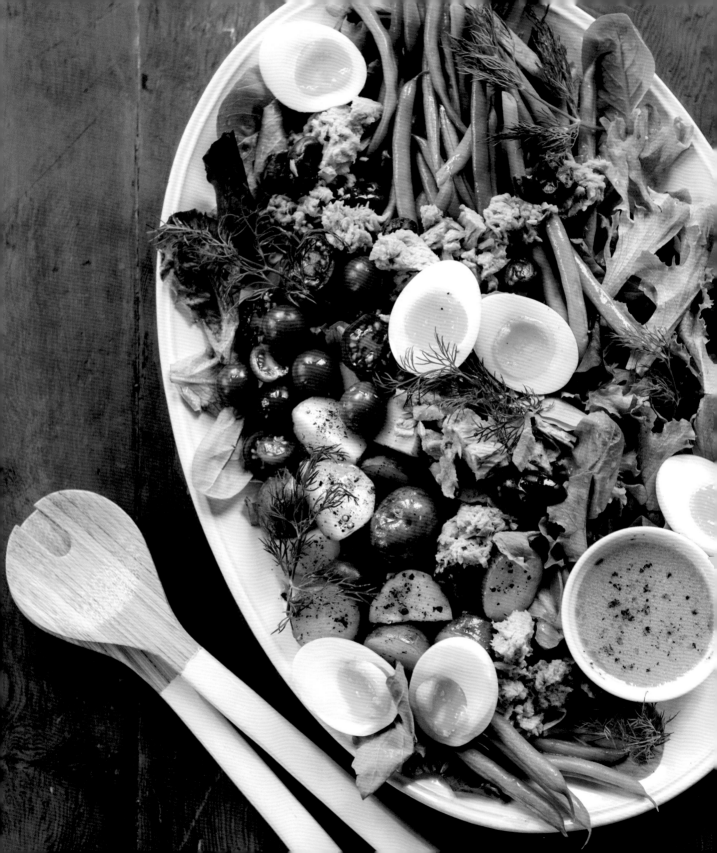

NIÇOISE SALAD

WHEAT-FREE
DAIRY-FREE
PESCATARIAN

Don't let its fancy French name fool you; this Niçoise Salad is packed with power thanks to ingredients like canned tuna and boiled eggs. Potatoes and olives help fill you up, and of course the gorgeous greens are loaded with the nutrients your body craves. I can't think of another salad that boasts as many health benefits but still tastes this good. A total must-try!

SERVINGS: **2**   PREP TIME: **10 MINUTES**   COOK TIME: **25 MINUTES**

---

2 medium red potatoes, washed and chopped

½ pound green beans, trimmed and halved

3 large eggs

¼ cup extra-virgin olive oil

3 tablespoons white wine vinegar

2 teaspoons grainy Dijon mustard

1 garlic clove, grated

Salt and freshly ground black pepper

6 cups mixed greens

1 cup halved cherry tomatoes

1 (5-ounce) can tuna, drained and flaked

¼ cup pitted Niçoise or Kalamata olives

Fresh dill, for garnish

IN a pot with a steamer insert, steam the red potatoes until they are tender, 10 to 12 minutes. Transfer the potatoes to a bowl lined with a paper towel and set them aside. In the same steamer, add the green beans and steam them until they are fork-tender, about 4 minutes. Transfer the green beans to a separate bowl lined with a paper towel.

IN a small saucepan, boil the eggs until they are cooked to your liking, 6 minutes for soft-boiled and 8 to 10 minutes for hard-boiled. Run the eggs under cold water until they are cool enough to handle. Peel them and cut them in half.

IN a small bowl, whisk together the olive oil, vinegar, mustard, garlic, and salt and pepper until well combined.

ARRANGE the mixed greens on a large serving platter. Top with the potatoes, green beans, tomatoes, eggs, tuna, and olives. Garnish with fresh dill.

DRESS and serve immediately or store the salad and the dressing separately in the refrigerator for up to 3 days.

simple swaps

The canned tuna in this recipe can be replaced with 5 ounces flaked cooked salmon or, for a vegetarian salad, removed entirely.

GREEK CHICKEN SOUP

DAIRY-FREE

I think we can all agree that chicken soup is the ultimate "comfort food," but I'll be honest, I didn't understand chicken soup's full potential until I tried the Greek version—avgolemono. This tasty twist on the classic uses lemon juice for tartness, eggs for richness, and loads of fresh herbs for even more amazing flavor. I promise that once you taste it, you'll never look at chicken soup the same way again.

SERVINGS: **4**   PREP TIME: **5 MINUTES**   COOK TIME: **25 TO 30 MINUTES**

---

1 tablespoon extra-virgin olive oil

1 medium yellow onion, diced

3 medium carrots, diced

3 celery stalks, diced

8 cups chicken broth, homemade (page 206) or store-bought

3 cups shredded cooked chicken

1 teaspoon fresh thyme leaves

1 bay leaf

1 cup orzo

2 large eggs

Juice of 1 lemon

2 tablespoons chopped fresh parsley

2 tablespoons chopped fresh dill

Salt and freshly ground black pepper

IN a large Dutch oven or soup pot, heat the olive oil over medium-high heat. Add the onion, carrots, and celery. Cook, stirring often, until they become tender, about 6 minutes. Add the broth, shredded chicken, thyme, and bay leaf. Bring the broth to a boil and add the orzo. Reduce the heat to medium and simmer until the orzo is cooked through, about 15 minutes.

IN a small heatproof bowl, whisk together the eggs and lemon juice. While whisking continuously, use a ladle to slowly add 1 cup of the hot broth to the egg mixture. (This process is called tempering and will prevent the raw eggs from scrambling when they're added to the hot soup.)

POUR the tempered egg mixture back into the soup pot and simmer for 5 minutes more. Stir in the fresh parsley and dill and season the soup with salt and pepper.

SERVE immediately or store in the refrigerator for up to 3 days.

simple swaps

To keep this soup gluten-free, you can replace the orzo with 1 cup uncooked white rice.

mix it up

To make this soup even more nutritious, stir in 4 cups chopped baby spinach during the last 2 minutes of cooking. Cook, stirring, until the spinach has wilted completely, then serve.

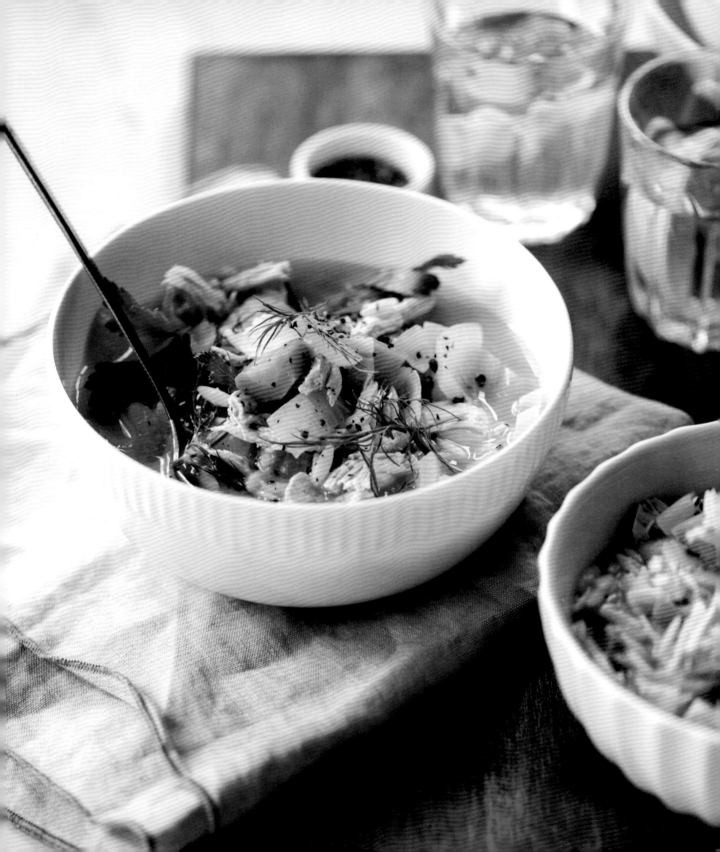

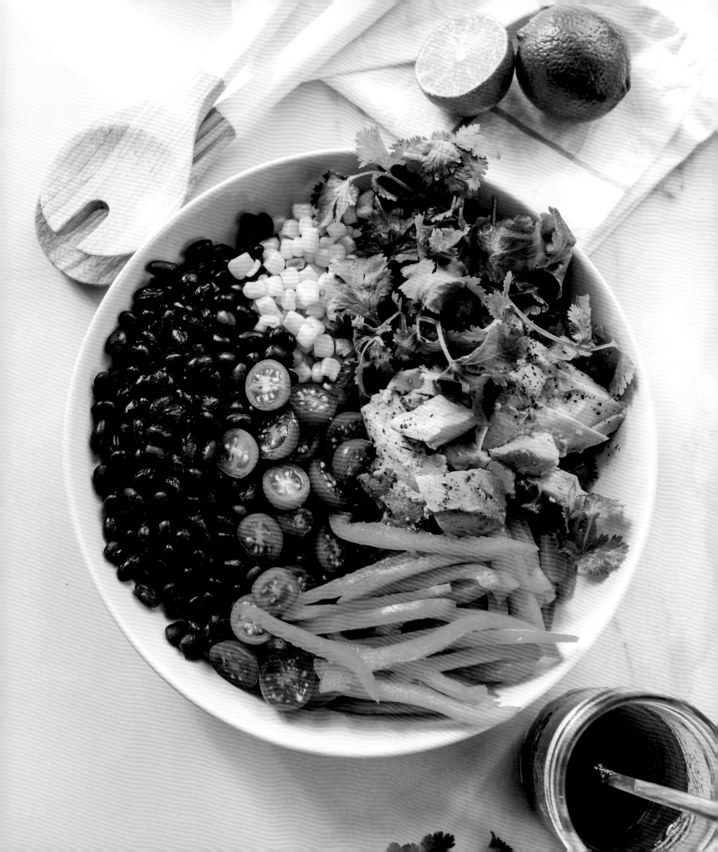

SOUTHWESTERN BLACK BEAN SALAD

VEGETARIAN

VEGAN

WHEAT-FREE

DAIRY-FREE

PESCATARIAN

There are few types of salad more filling than a fiber-rich bean salad, and this delicious black bean version with its zesty, Southwestern-inspired flavors is sure to become a lunch staple. This dish can be made during your Sunday meal prep and enjoyed throughout the week, so feel free to double the recipe.

SERVINGS: **2**   PREP TIME: **10 MINUTES**

---

2 tablespoons vegetable oil

Grated zest and juice of 2 limes

1 teaspoon chili powder

½ teaspoon ground cumin

Salt and freshly ground black pepper

1 (15-ounce) can black beans, drained and rinsed

1 cup fresh or frozen corn kernels

1 orange bell pepper, diced

1 cup halved cherry tomatoes

1 avocado, diced

¼ cup chopped fresh cilantro

IN a small bowl, whisk together the oil, lime zest, lime juice, chili powder, cumin, and salt and pepper until well combined.

IN a large bowl, combine the black beans, corn, bell pepper, tomatoes, avocado, and cilantro. (If you plan on making this ahead of time, do not add the avocado until just before serving.) Pour the dressing over the salad and toss until everything is evenly coated.

SERVE immediately or store in the refrigerator for up to 4 days.

mix it up

Replace the dressing in this recipe with ¼ cup Salsa Verde (page 215). To add more protein to this dish, stir in 1 cup shredded cooked chicken.

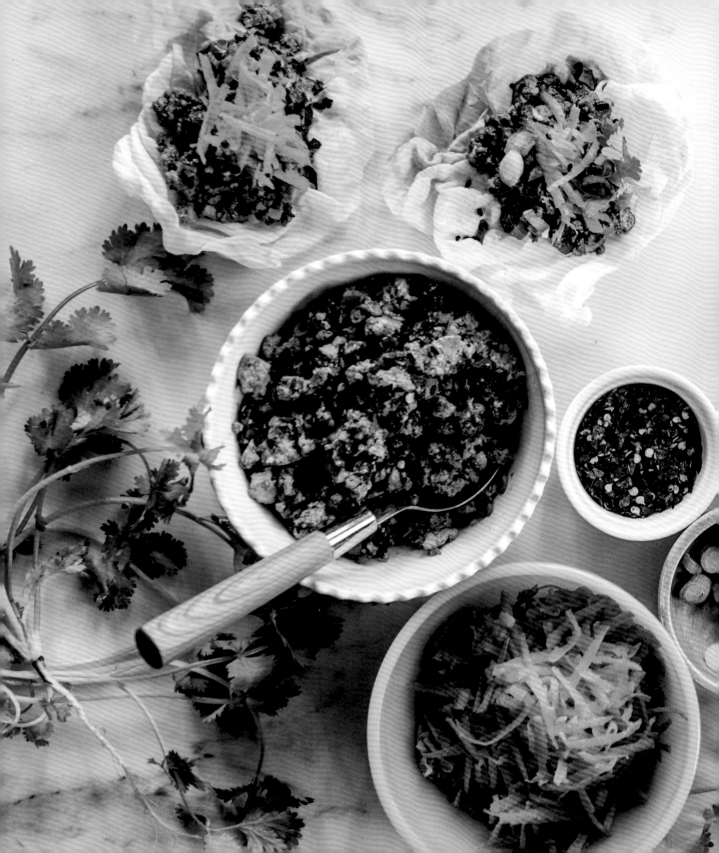

LETTUCE WRAPS

Lettuce Wraps are an amazing way to lighten up your lunch. If your goal is to go gluten-free or just to trim a few extra calories, then these crisp, refreshing wraps are the way to go. When it comes to the lettuce itself, you want something that will hold its shape when you pick it up—I prefer Bibb lettuce, but romaine also works well. Here are three filling ideas I love . . .

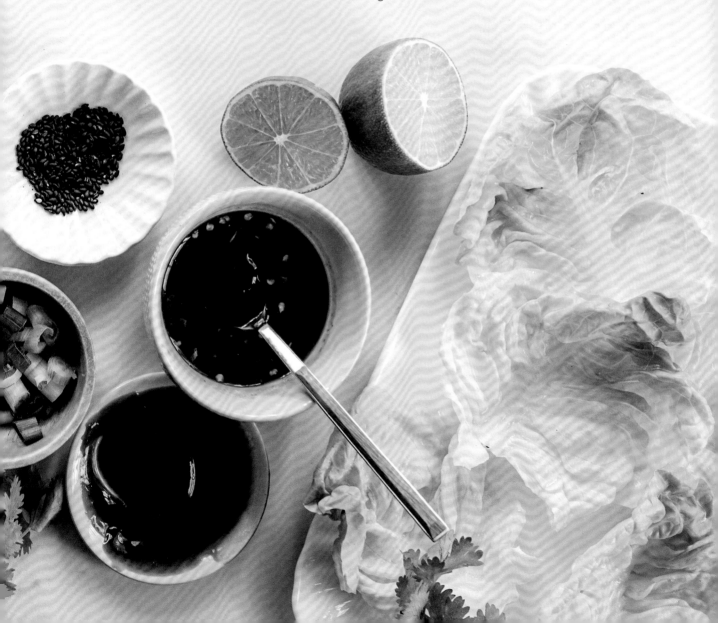

CHICKEN CLUB LETTUCE WRAPS

SERVINGS: **1**   PREP TIME: **5 MINUTES**

1 cup shredded cooked
   chicken

1 avocado, diced

½ cup halved cherry tomatoes

2 bacon slices, cooked and
   chopped (optional)

1 tablespoon ranch dressing

4 or 5 Bibb or small romaine
   lettuce leaves

IN a medium bowl, combine the chicken, avocado, tomato, bacon (if using), and ranch dressing. Gently toss until everything is evenly coated in the dressing.

SPOON the mixture into the center of each lettuce leaf (I use an ice cream scoop for this).

ENJOY immediately or store the filling in the fridge for up to 3 days and assemble just before eating.

mix it up

To make a Cobb salad wrap, replace the ranch dressing with 1 tablespoon Blue Cheese Dressing (page 227) and add 1 diced hard-boiled egg.

MANGO SHRIMP LETTUCE WRAPS

SERVINGS: **1**   PREP TIME: **5 MINUTES**

1 cup chopped cooked shrimp

½ cup finely diced mango

¼ cup finely diced cucumber

2 tablespoons minced red onion

1 tablespoon chopped fresh cilantro

Juice of 1 lime

½ red chile, minced (optional)

Salt and freshly ground black pepper

4 or 5 Bibb or small romaine lettuce leaves

IN a medium bowl, combine the shrimp, mango, cucumber, onion, cilantro, lime juice, chile (if using), and salt and pepper. Gently toss until well mixed.

SPOON the mixture into the center of each lettuce leaf (I use an ice cream scoop for this).

ENJOY immediately or store the filling in the fridge for up to 3 days and assemble just before eating.

simple swaps

You can always swap out the mango for some finely diced pineapple.

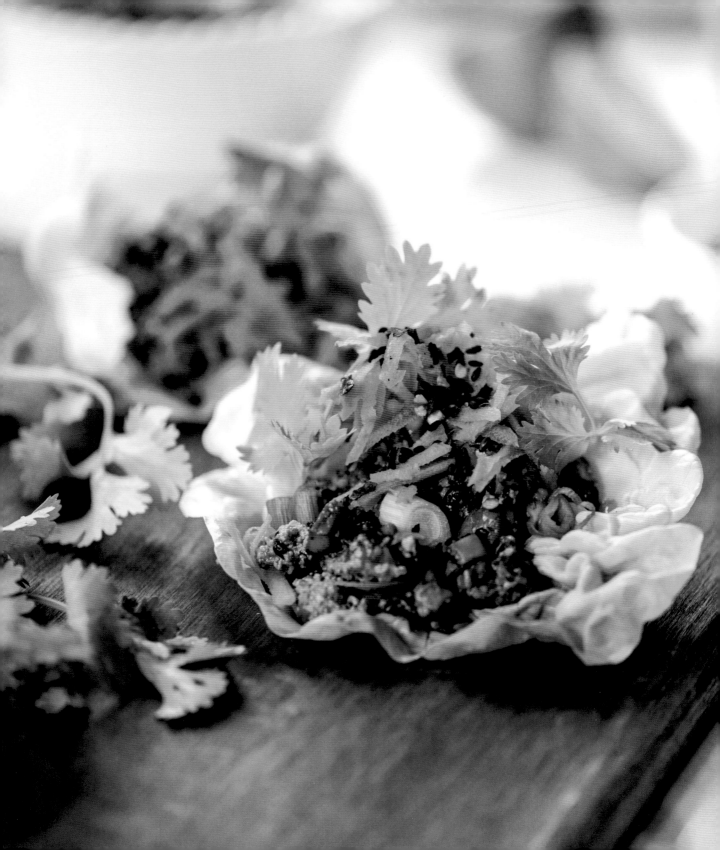

VEGAN CHICK'N LETTUCE WRAPS

VEGETARIAN

VEGAN

DAIRY-FREE

PESCATARIAN

SERVINGS: **1** PREP TIME: **5 MINUTES** COOK TIME: **10 MINUTES**

1 tablespoon sesame oil

½ cup finely diced cremini mushrooms

¼ cup finely diced yellow onion

1 garlic clove, minced

½ teaspoon grated fresh ginger

1 cup crumbled extra-firm tofu

2 tablespoons hoisin sauce

1 tablespoon soy sauce

1 tablespoon rice vinegar

½ teaspoon red pepper flakes (optional)

4 or 5 Bibb or small romaine lettuce leaves

¼ cup shredded carrot, for garnish

1 green onion, sliced, for garnish

Fresh cilantro, for garnish

Black sesame seeds, for garnish

IN a large wok or nonstick skillet, heat the sesame oil over medium-high heat. Add the mushrooms and onion and cook, stirring, until they have softened, about 4 minutes. Stir in the garlic and ginger and cook for 30 seconds. Add the tofu, hoisin sauce, soy sauce, vinegar, and red pepper flakes (if using) and cook, stirring often, for 2 to 3 minutes more.

SPOON the mixture into the center of each lettuce leaf (I use an ice cream scoop for this). Top each with some shredded carrot, green onion, cilantro, and sesame seeds.

ENJOY immediately or let cool completely and store the filling in the fridge for up to 4 days. Assemble just before eating.

BBQ CHICKEN & PINEAPPLE SALAD

WHEAT-FREE

This bright, fresh summer salad is bursting with flavor thanks to the tangy grilled pineapple and smoky-sweet BBQ chicken. I've topped it with savory ham and a cool, creamy ranch dressing to balance all the flavors. Find a seat on the patio, because this deliciousness is best enjoyed in the sunshine.

SERVINGS: **2**   PREP TIME: **5 MINUTES**   COOK TIME: **20 MINUTES**

---

2 small boneless, skinless chicken breasts

2 teaspoons vegetable oil

Salt and freshly ground black pepper

½ pineapple, cored and sliced into rings

3 tablespoons barbecue sauce

4 cups chopped romaine lettuce

1 cup halved cherry tomatoes

½ cup chopped deli ham

¼ red onion, finely sliced

¼ cup ranch dressing

Fresh parsley, for garnish

HEAT a grill to medium-high.

BRUSH the chicken breasts with the vegetable oil and season both sides liberally with salt and pepper.

ARRANGE the pineapple slices on one side of the grill and the chicken breasts on the other. Cook the pineapple until it has developed significant grill marks on one side, about 6 minutes. Use tongs to turn it and cook until grill marks develop on the other side, 4 to 6 minutes. Remove the pineapple from the grill and set it aside.

MEANWHILE, cook the chicken until the first side has developed grill marks and releases easily from the grill grates, about 8 minutes. Turn the chicken and cook on the second side for 6 minutes.

REDUCE the grill heat to medium. Brush the chicken with barbecue sauce on both sides and grill for an additional 2 minutes per side, or until a meat thermometer inserted into each breast registers 165°F. Remove the chicken from the grill and let cool for 5 minutes before slicing.

IN a large serving bowl, layer the lettuce, grilled pineapple, tomatoes, ham, and onion. Arrange the sliced chicken on top and finish with the ranch dressing.

SERVE immediately, garnished with fresh parsley, or store in the refrigerator for up to 3 days.

simple swaps

- To keep this dish dairy-free, simply replace the ranch dressing with ¼ cup White Wine Vinaigrette (page 224).
- The BBQ chicken in this recipe can be replaced with grilled shrimp or tofu.

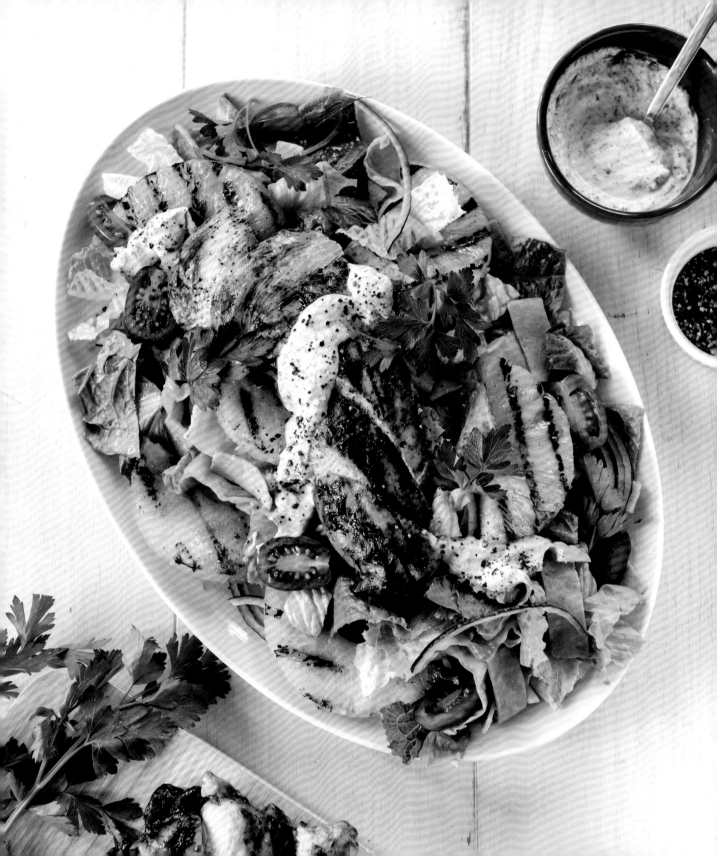

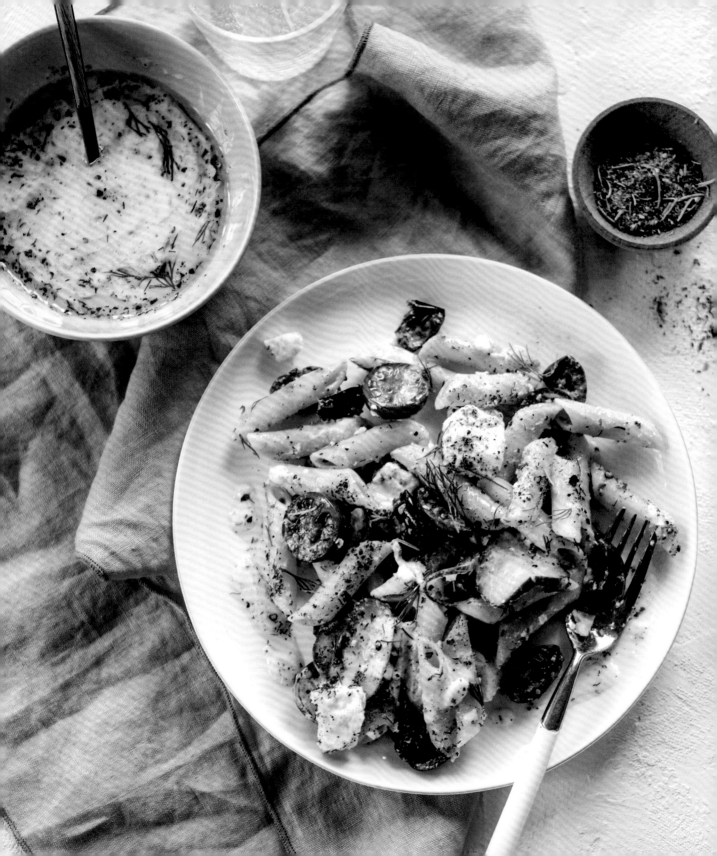

CREAMY GREEK PASTA SALAD

VEGETARIAN
PESCATARIAN

This Creamy Greek Pasta Salad will elevate you to the status of lunch legend among your colleagues. It's rich, creamy, and very filling, but also includes lots of healthy ingredients you can feel really good about. And it tastes just as good as it looks. You're welcome!

SERVINGS: **4**   PREP TIME: **5 MINUTES**   COOK TIME: **10 MINUTES**

Salt

1 pound penne pasta

½ English cucumber, diced

½ cup halved cherry tomatoes

¼ cup sliced pitted Kalamata olives

¼ cup crumbled feta cheese

1 cup Tzatziki Sauce (page 222)

1 tablespoon Greek Seasoning (page 230)

Ground black pepper

1 tablespoon olive oil (optional)

Fresh dill, for garnish

IN a large pot, bring 4 quarts water to a rolling boil over high heat. Salt the water generously and add the pasta. Reduce the heat to medium-high and cook the pasta, stirring, until al dente, about 10 minutes. Drain the pasta in a colander and let cool.

IN a large bowl, combine the cooled pasta, cucumber, tomatoes, olives, and feta and toss well. Add the tzatziki and Greek Seasoning and season with salt and pepper. Toss until everything is well coated. If the dressing needs to be thinned, add the olive oil.

ENJOY immediately, garnished with fresh dill, or store in the refrigerator for up to 4 days, though I always recommend dressing the pasta just before eating it.

mix it up

Add even more wonderful Mediterranean flavor with ½ cup chopped artichoke hearts, ¼ cup chopped roasted red peppers, and 2 tablespoons capers.

CHICKPEA & AVOCADO SMASH SANDWICH

VEGETARIAN

PESCATARIAN

VEGAN

DAIRY-FREE

Picking a favorite recipe is like picking a favorite child—you're not supposed to do it. But if I had to, this might just be the one. It's hard to believe that such a simple combination of ingredients can make such an impact, but this sandwich does just that. And as if that wasn't enough, it's also completely vegan. What's not to love?

SERVINGS: **2**   PREP TIME: **10 MINUTES**

1 (15-ounce) can chickpeas, drained and rinsed

¼ cup finely diced red onion

¼ cup finely diced dill pickles

2 tablespoons chopped fresh dill

1 tablespoon dill pickle brine (from the pickle jar)

1 tablespoon extra-virgin olive oil

2 teaspoons grainy Dijon mustard

Salt and freshly ground black pepper

1 ripe avocado

Juice of ½ lemon

4 thick slices sourdough bread

Arugula, for serving

IN a large bowl, combine the chickpeas, onion, pickles, dill, pickle brine, olive oil, and mustard. Season the mixture liberally with salt and pepper. Stir well.

IN a second bowl, mash the avocado with a fork. Stir in the lemon juice.

ASSEMBLE the sandwiches by spreading half the avocado mash on one slice of bread and then piling half the chickpea mixture on top. Finish with arugula and another slice of bread. Repeat to make a second sandwich.

ENJOY immediately or store the chickpea mixture in the refrigerator for up to 4 days and assemble the sandwiches just before eating.

simple swaps

If you're not a fan of chickpeas, replace them with navy or cannellini beans.

mix it up

Instead of using bread and making sandwiches, keep this gluten-free by serving the chickpeas and avocado over baby spinach or in lettuce wraps.

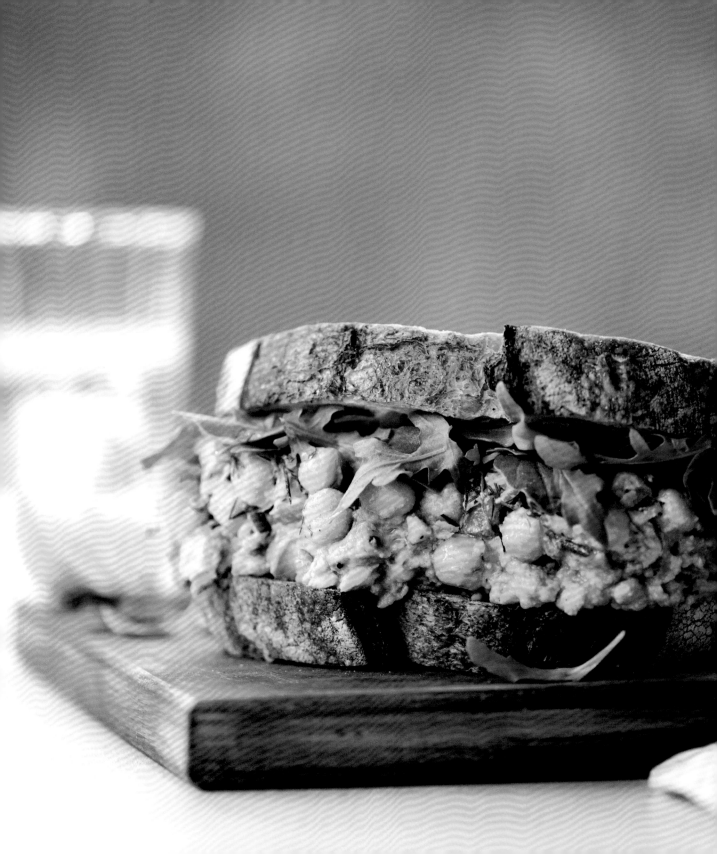

TUNA POKE BOWL

DAIRY-FREE

PESCATARIAN

Poke (pronounced *poh-kay*) has been a huge food trend for a couple of years now, and it's not hard to understand why. It's healthy, filling, and, above all else, really tasty when prepared well. When you're selecting your fish for this dish, it's very important to use sushi-grade tuna. Your local fishmonger is the best place to find it. Seaweed salad can typically be found in the prepared foods section of most large supermarkets.

SERVINGS: **1**   PREP TIME: **5 MINUTES**

---

1 tablespoon soy sauce

1 teaspoon rice vinegar

1 teaspoon sesame oil

1 cup cooked brown rice

4 ounces sushi-grade tuna, diced

½ cup prepared seaweed salad

¼ avocado, sliced

1 tablespoon pickled ginger

1 green onion, chopped

½ teaspoon black sesame seeds

IN a small bowl, whisk together the soy sauce, vinegar, and sesame oil.

IN a serving bowl, layer the rice, tuna, seaweed salad, avocado, and pickled ginger.

POUR the dressing over the ingredients and top the bowl with the green onion and sesame seeds.

SERVE immediately.

simple swaps

- The sushi-grade tuna in this recipe can be swapped out for sushi-grade salmon instead.
- If you're not comfortable consuming raw fish, replace the tuna with 6 large cooked shrimp or ¾ cup sautéed mushrooms.

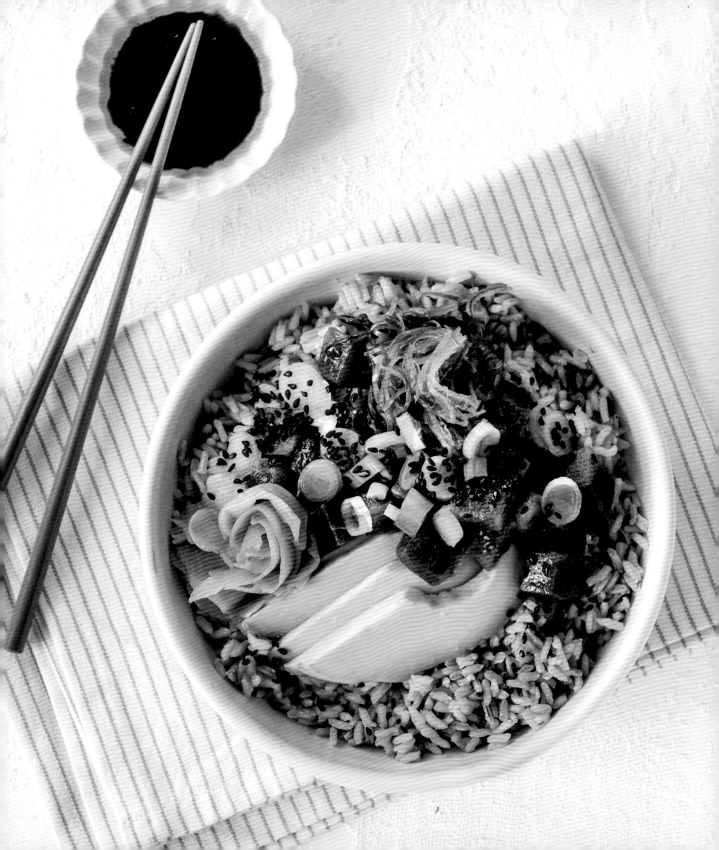

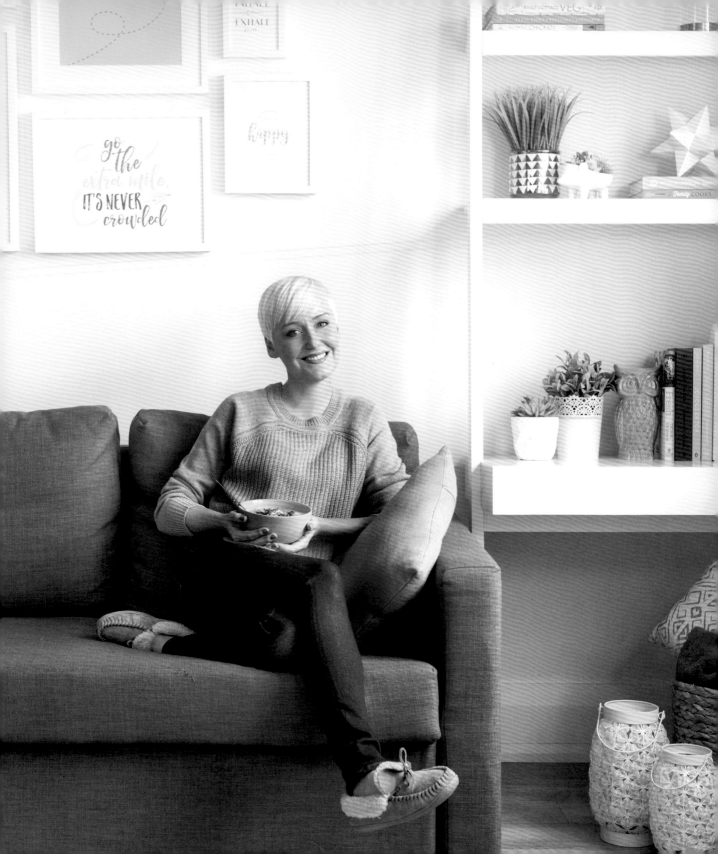

FISH TACO BOWL

Fish tacos are actually one of my all-time favorite foods, but—let's be honest—they don't exactly travel well, so I created my Fish Taco Bowl. It's got all the goodness of traditional fish tacos but can be easily transported to work. And trust me, this dish will make you the envy of the lunchroom.

SERVINGS: **1**   PREP TIME: **5 MINUTES**

1 cup cooked long-grain and wild rice blend

½ cup shredded red cabbage

½ cup canned black beans, drained and rinsed

½ cup Pineapple Salsa (page 217)

1 (4-ounce) tilapia fillet, cooked and flaked

¼ avocado, sliced

Lime wedges, for serving

Fresh cilantro, for serving

IN a serving bowl, layer the wild rice, cabbage, black beans, and pineapple salsa. Top with the tilapia.

JUST before eating, add the avocado and dress the salad with freshly squeezed lime juice and cilantro.

SERVE immediately or store in the refrigerator for up to 3 days.

simple swaps

- The tilapia in this recipe can be replaced with cooked shrimp.
- If you want to keep this bowl grain-free, go ahead and replace the wild rice with baby spinach or mixed greens.

mix it up

To turn this goodness back into tacos, divide the ingredients among 4 corn tortillas.

VEGAN POWER BOWL

This Vegan Power Bowl is sure to satisfy, thanks to lots of protein and fiber from healthy ingredients like chickpeas and quinoa. Even if you're not vegan, this is a delicious way to get more veggies into your diet and the perfect way to celebrate Meatless Monday.

VEGETARIAN
VEGAN
WHEAT-FREE
DAIRY-FREE
PESCATARIAN

SERVINGS: **1**   PREP TIME: **5 MINUTES**

---

2 cups finely chopped kale leaves

2 tablespoons Balsamic Vinaigrette (page 226)

½ cup shredded red cabbage

½ cup roasted sweet potato cubes (see below)

½ cup canned chickpeas, drained and rinsed

½ cup cooked quinoa (see page 34)

2 tablespoons chopped almonds

IN a large bowl, toss the kale with 1 tablespoon of the vinaigrette until well coated.

TRANSFER the kale to a serving bowl and layer in the cabbage, sweet potato, chickpeas, and quinoa. Top with the almonds and dress with the remaining 1 tablespoon vinaigrette.

SERVE immediately or store in the refrigerator for up to 4 days.

simple swaps

- The kale in the recipe can be replaced with any nutritious greens like spinach, Swiss chard, or romaine lettuce.
- To keep this dish nut-free, replace the chopped almonds with pumpkin seeds (pepitas) or sunflower seeds.

HOW TO ROAST SWEET POTATOES

Preheat the oven to 400°F. Peel the sweet potato and chop it into ½-inch cubes. Arrange the cubes on a baking sheet. Toss them with 2 teaspoons olive oil and season with salt and pepper. Bake, turning once, until the sweet potato cubes are tender, 25 to 30 minutes.

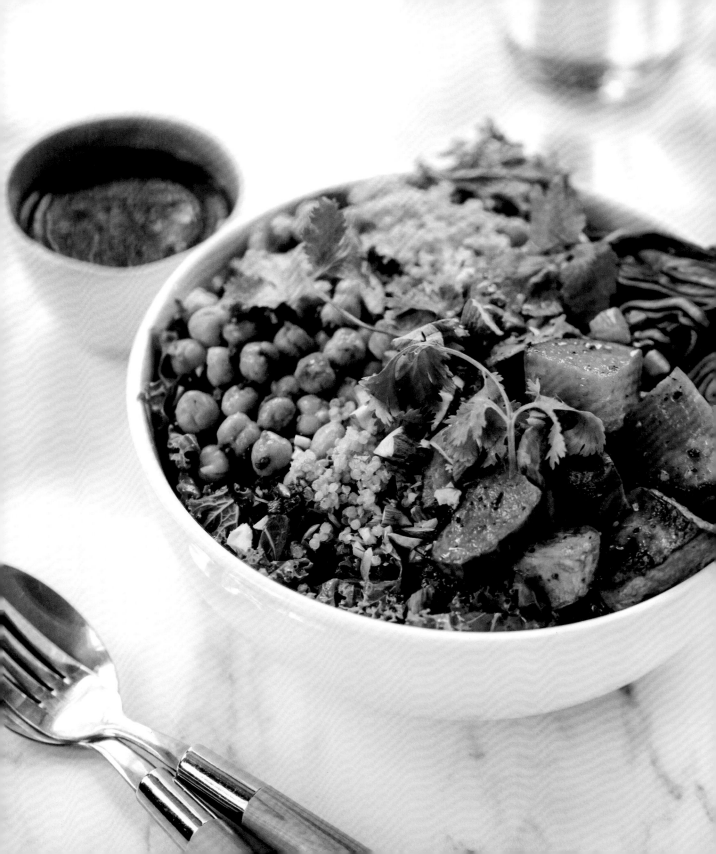

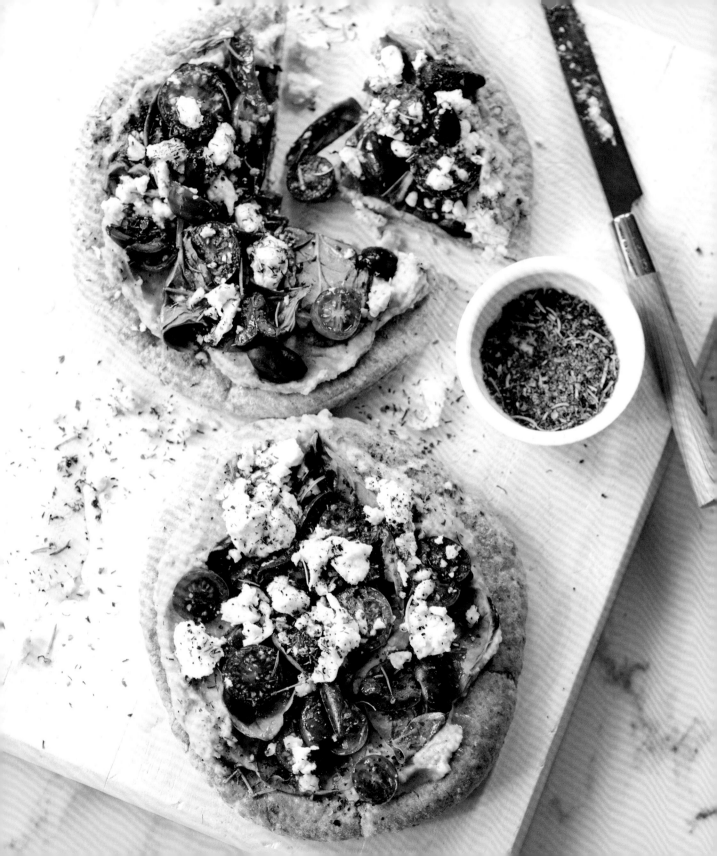

PITA PIZZAS

When it's lunchtime and I'm at my laziest, Pita Pizzas are the answer. They can be prepped in a flash and cook just as quickly. If you're making them at the office, I always recommend opting for the toaster oven over the microwave for best results.

MEDITERRANEAN PITA PIZZAS

VEGETARIAN

PESCATARIAN

SERVINGS: **2**   PREP TIME: **5 MINUTES**   COOK TIME: **10 MINUTES**

½ cup hummus, homemade (page 221) or store-bought

2 small whole wheat pitas

½ cup chopped baby spinach (¾ to 1 ounce)

½ cup halved cherry tomatoes

2 tablespoons chopped pitted Kalamata olives

2 tablespoons crumbled feta cheese

1 teaspoon Greek Seasoning (page 230)

PREHEAT the oven or toaster oven to 375°F.

SPREAD a layer of hummus over each pita. Top evenly with the baby spinach, tomatoes, olives, and feta. Sprinkle with the Greek Seasoning.

ARRANGE the pitas on a baking sheet and bake for 8 to 10 minutes, until the spinach has wilted and the cheese is just golden.

ENJOY immediately.

TURKEY CRAN-BRIE PITA PIZZAS

SERVINGS: **2**   PREP TIME: **5 MINUTES**   COOK TIME: **10 MINUTES**

6 slices oven-roasted turkey breast

2 small whole wheat pitas

4 to 6 ounces Brie cheese, thinly sliced

¼ cup cranberry sauce

½ teaspoon fresh thyme leaves

PREHEAT the oven or toaster oven to 375°F.

ARRANGE 3 slices of the turkey on each pita and then top evenly with the Brie, cranberry sauce, and thyme.

ARRANGE the pitas on a baking sheet and bake for 8 to 10 minutes, until the Brie has melted completely and the pizzas are heated through.

ENJOY immediately.

TUNA MELT PITA PIZZAS

SERVINGS: **2** PREP TIME: **5 MINUTES** COOK TIME: **10 MINUTES**

1 (5-ounce) can tuna, drained and flaked

1 cup chopped baby spinach (1½ to 2 ounces)

2 tablespoons mayonnaise

2 green onions, thinly sliced

Salt and freshly ground black pepper

2 whole wheat pitas

½ cup shredded sharp cheddar cheese

Chopped fresh parsley, for garnish

PREHEAT the oven or toaster oven to 375°F.

IN a medium bowl, combine the tuna, spinach, mayonnaise, green onions, and salt and pepper. Stir well.

DIVIDE the mixture between the pitas and spread it evenly. Top each with half the cheese.

ARRANGE the pitas on a baking sheet and bake for 8 to 10 minutes, until the cheese has melted and the pizzas are heated through. Garnish with the parsley.

ENJOY immediately.

VEGGIE FRIED QUINOA

VEGETARIAN

DAIRY-FREE

PESCATARIAN

Of all the dishes I've shared on my YouTube channel over the years, Veggie Fried Quinoa is one of the most popular among aspiring home cooks. It's healthy, versatile, and effortless to whip up when you need something quick but satisfying. To make things easier, I always cook some quinoa during my Sunday meal prep so it's ready to go when I need it throughout the week.

SERVINGS: **4**   PREP TIME: **5 MINUTES**   COOK TIME: **15 MINUTES**

---

1 tablespoon vegetable oil

1 small yellow onion, diced

1 cup frozen peas and carrots

1 garlic clove, minced

2 large eggs, beaten

3 cups cooked quinoa (see page 34)

3 tablespoons soy sauce

2 teaspoons sriracha sauce (optional)

2 green onions, chopped

IN a large wok or nonstick skillet, heat the vegetable oil over medium-high heat. Add the onion and cook, stirring often, until soft and translucent, 3 to 4 minutes. Add the frozen peas and carrots and cook, stirring, for 2 to 3 minutes. Add the garlic and cook, stirring, for 30 seconds. Use a wooden spoon or rubber spatula to move the vegetable mixture to one side of the pan.

ON the other side of the pan, pour in the beaten eggs and cook, stirring continuously, until they are scrambled, 1 to 2 minutes. Once the eggs are scrambled, mix them with the vegetables and then add the quinoa, soy sauce, and sriracha (if using). Cook, stirring continuously, until the quinoa is heated through, 2 to 3 minutes. Turn off the heat and stir in the green onions.

SERVE immediately or let cool completely and store in the refrigerator for 3 to 4 days. It can be enjoyed cold or reheated.

mix it up

For the veggies, I've kept it simple with just frozen peas and carrots, but you can get creative by adding frozen green beans, corn, or shelled edamame. If you're feeling adventurous, you can even try ½ cup diced pineapple for a touch of sweetness.

To amp up the protein in this dish, try adding 1 cup shredded cooked chicken or ½ pound cooked shrimp when you add the quinoa.

simple swaps

- For those of you who aren't fond of quinoa, you can certainly use cooked rice instead. And if you're looking for a lower-carb option, try cooked cauliflower rice.
- To make this recipe gluten-free, swap out the soy sauce for some gluten-free tamari.

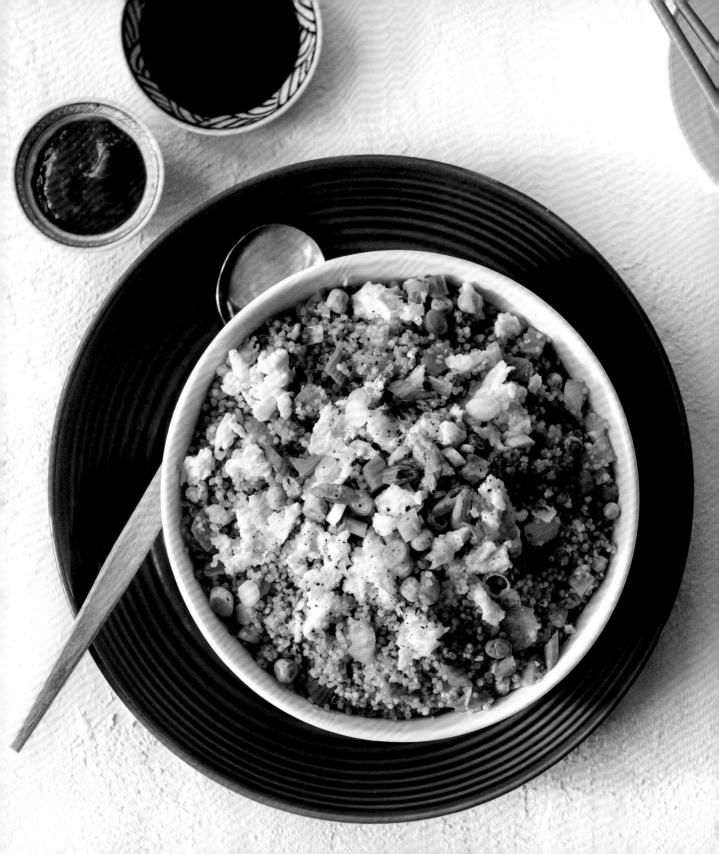

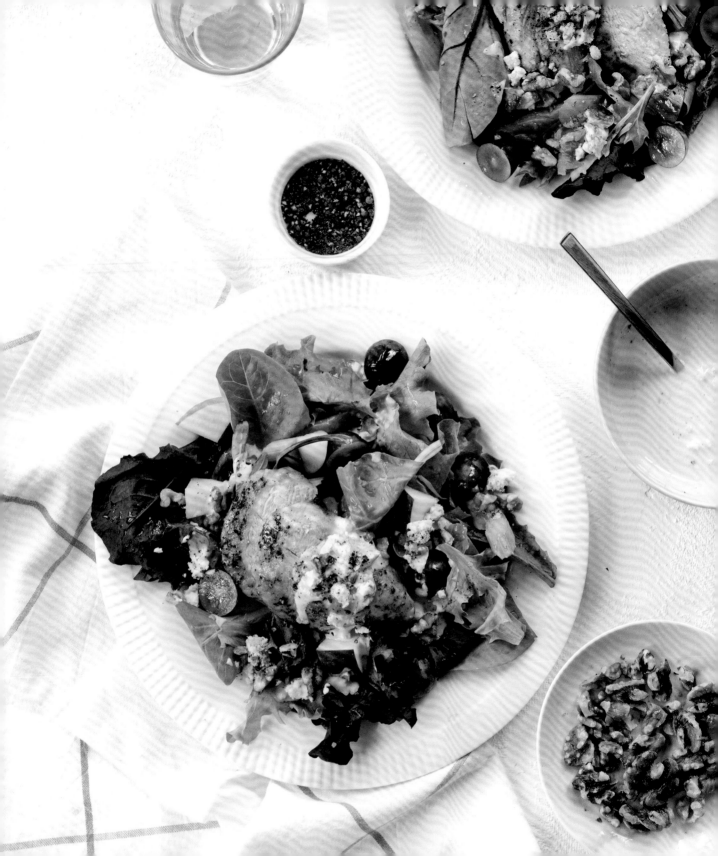

WALDORF SALAD

The Waldorf Salad has a rich history dating back to the late 1800s, when it was first served at the Waldorf Hotel in New York City. It has since fallen out of favor, but I think that's a real shame because the flavors are just so timeless. I really love reviving a classic, so I've added a few tasty twists here. I hope you enjoy it as much as I do.

SERVINGS: **1**   PREP TIME: **5 MINUTES**   COOK TIME: **25 MINUTES**

---

1 boneless, skinless chicken breast

Salt and freshly ground black pepper

2 cups mixed greens

½ apple, cored and diced

½ cup halved red grapes

¼ cup chopped celery

2 tablespoons chopped walnuts

2 tablespoons Blue Cheese Dressing (page 227)

PREHEAT the oven to 375°F.

SEASON the chicken breast liberally on both sides with salt and pepper. Transfer to a baking dish and bake until a meat thermometer inserted into the chicken breast registers 165°F, about 25 minutes. Remove the chicken and let cool for 5 minutes before slicing.

IN a large serving bowl, layer the mixed greens, apple, grapes, celery, and walnuts. Add the sliced chicken breast. Just before serving, top the salad with the Blue Cheese Dressing.

SERVE immediately, or store the undressed salad in the refrigerator for up to 3 days and dress just before serving.

simple swaps

For those of you who aren't fans of blue cheese, you can always swap it out for ranch dressing instead.

mix it up

For a flavorful take on chicken salad, combine shredded cooked chicken, apple, grapes, celery, and walnuts and toss it all with blue cheese dressing. The chicken salad can be served on bread or in lettuce wraps.

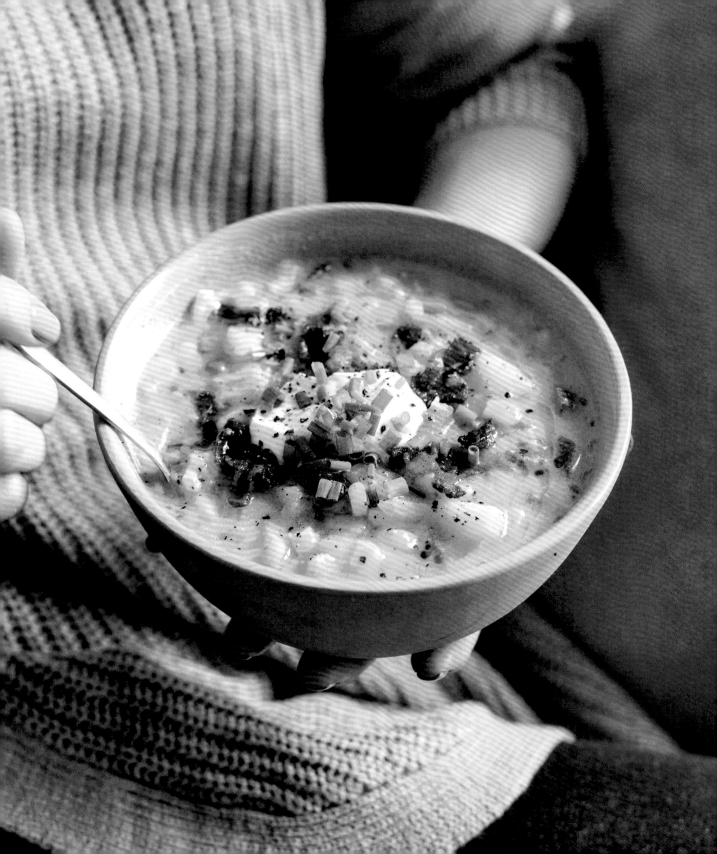

SMOKY CORN CHOWDER

When it comes to comfort food, this corn chowder simply can't be beat. It's the perfect balance of sweet, savory, spicy, and smoky thanks to the addition of chipotle peppers. With an abundance of fiber-rich ingredients like corn and potatoes, this soup is hearty and satisfying. Pair it with a fresh mixed green salad, and lunch is served.

SERVINGS: **4**   PREP TIME: **10 MINUTES**   COOK TIME: **35 MINUTES**

---

2 bacon slices, chopped

1 yellow onion, diced

2 celery stalks, diced

1 red bell pepper, diced

1 garlic clove, minced

2 canned chipotle peppers in adobo sauce, minced

3 cups chicken broth, homemade (page 206) or store-bought

3 cups fresh or frozen corn kernels

2 russet potatoes, peeled and diced

1 cup 2% milk

1 tablespoon flour

2 tablespoons water

Salt and freshly ground black pepper

Sour cream, for serving

Minced fresh chives, for serving

IN a large soup pot or Dutch oven, cook the bacon over medium-high heat, stirring occasionally, until crispy and golden, 6 to 8 minutes. Use a slotted spoon to transfer the bacon to a plate lined with paper towels. Remove all but 1 tablespoon of the bacon fat from the pot.

TO the same pot, add the onion, celery, and bell pepper and cook, stirring, until they begin to soften, 4 to 5 minutes. Add the garlic and chipotle peppers and cook, stirring, for 30 seconds. Add the broth, corn, potatoes, milk, and cooked bacon. Bring the mixture to a simmer, then reduce the heat to medium and cook until the potatoes are tender, about 15 minutes.

IN a small bowl, stir together the flour and water. Add the flour mixture to the pot and cook, stirring continuously, until the soup has thickened slightly, 2 to 3 minutes. Season with salt and pepper.

SERVE hot, with a dollop of sour cream and some chives, or let cool completely and store in the refrigerator for 3 to 4 days or in the freezer for up to 3 months.

simple swaps

To keep this soup vegetarian, skip the bacon and use 1 tablespoon vegetable oil to cook the vegetables instead. Add 1 tablespoon smoked paprika for additional flavor.

EASY CHEESY QUESADILLAS

Quesadillas are adored by kids and adults alike, which is what makes them such a family-friendly lunch idea. They're effortless to make and can be dolled up with so many different flavor combinations that even the pickiest eaters can't resist. Here are a few of my favorite quesadilla recipes . . .

BLACK BEAN & CORN QUESADILLAS

VEGETARIAN

PESCATARIAN

SERVINGS: **2**   PREP TIME: **5 MINUTES**   COOK TIME: **10 MINUTES**

4 large whole wheat tortillas

¾ cup shredded cheddar cheese

½ cup canned black beans, drained and rinsed

½ cup fresh or frozen corn kernels

½ cup finely diced red bell pepper

1 tablespoon chopped green onion

½ teaspoon chili powder

Hot sauce

Salsa Fresca (page 214) and Homemade Guacamole (page 218), for serving

HEAT a large skillet over medium-high heat. Place one tortilla in the skillet and layer on 3 tablespoons of the cheese. Top with ¼ cup each of the black beans, corn, and bell pepper, half the green onion, ¼ teaspoon of the chili powder, and some hot sauce. Add 3 tablespoons more cheese and top with a second tortilla.

COOK until the cheese begins to melt, 2 to 3 minutes. Carefully flip the quesadilla and cook until all the cheese has melted, 1 to 2 minutes more. Remove the quesadilla from the skillet and repeat with the remaining ingredients to make a second quesadilla.

CUT the quesadillas into quarters and serve immediately, with salsa and guacamole.

simple swaps

Replace the flour tortillas with corn tortillas to keep this dish gluten-free.

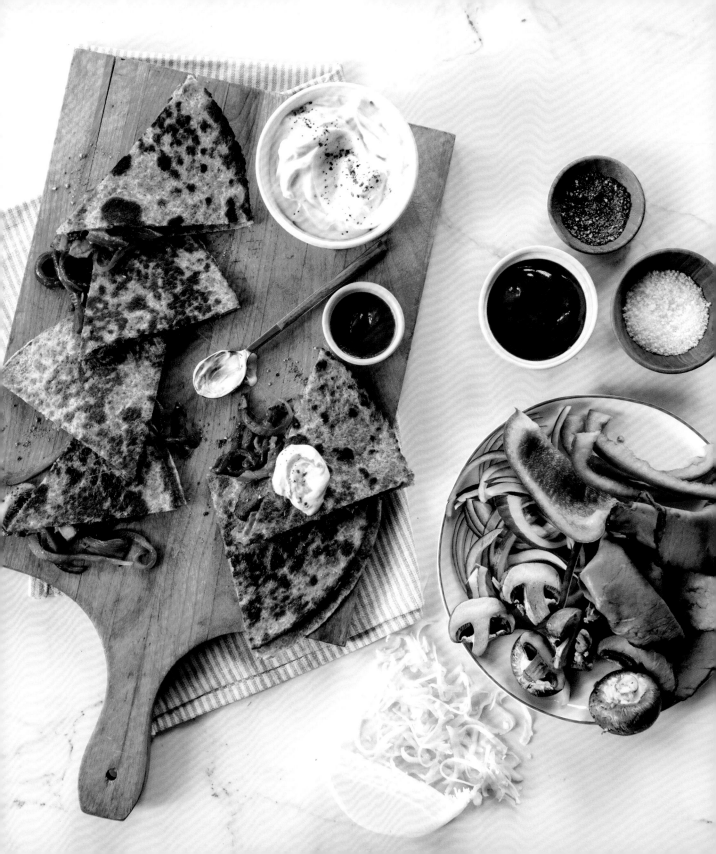

CAPRESE CHICKEN QUESADILLAS

SERVINGS: **2**   PREP TIME: **5 MINUTES**   COOK TIME: **10 MINUTES**

1 cup shredded cooked chicken

2 tablespoons Pesto Sauce (page 210)

4 large whole wheat tortillas

¾ cup shredded mozzarella cheese

½ cup finely chopped tomatoes

Tomato Sauce (page 208), for serving

IN a small bowl, toss the chicken in the pesto sauce until it's evenly coated.

HEAT a large skillet over medium-high heat. Place one tortilla in the skillet and layer on 3 tablespoons of the cheese. Top with half the pesto chicken and half the tomatoes. Add 3 tablespoons more cheese and top with a second tortilla.

COOK until the cheese begins to melt, 2 to 3 minutes. Carefully flip the quesadilla and cook until all the cheese has melted, 1 to 2 minutes more. Remove the quesadilla from the skillet and repeat with the remaining ingredients to make a second quesadilla.

CUT the quesadillas into quarters and serve immediately, with tomato sauce for dipping.

simple swaps

Try replacing the tomatoes with some finely diced roasted red peppers.

PHILLY CHEESE QUESADILLAS

SERVINGS: **2**   PREP TIME: **5 MINUTES**   COOK TIME: **15 MINUTES**

2 teaspoons vegetable oil

½ cup sliced cremini mushrooms

½ green bell pepper, thinly sliced

¼ cup sliced red onion

1 tablespoon steak sauce

½ teaspoon hot sauce (optional)

¼ teaspoon garlic powder

Salt and freshly ground black pepper

4 large whole wheat tortillas

¾ cup shredded provolone cheese

6 slices deli roast beef, chopped

Sour cream, for serving.

HEAT the oil in a skillet over medium-high heat. Add the mushrooms, bell pepper, and onion. Cook, stirring often, until softened, about 6 minutes. Add the steak sauce, hot sauce (if using), garlic powder, salt, and pepper and cook, stirring, for 30 seconds. Transfer the mixture to a bowl and wipe out the pan with a paper towel.

RETURN the skillet to the stove over medium-high heat. Place one tortilla in the skillet and layer with 3 tablespoons of the cheese. Top with half the roast beef and half the mushroom mixture. Add 3 tablespoons more cheese and top with a second tortilla.

COOK until the cheese begins to melt, 2 to 3 minutes. Carefully flip the quesadilla and cook until all the cheese has melted, 1 to 2 minutes more. Remove the quesadilla from the skillet and repeat with the remaining ingredients to make a second quesadilla.

CUT the quesadillas into quarters and serve immediately, with sour cream on the side for dipping.

simple swaps

Skip the roast beef to make this quesadilla vegetarian.

MEDITERRANEAN TUNA SALAD

This light, fresh, and flavorful take on tuna salad is sure to become a lunch favorite. Instead of heavy mayo, I've used a tangy vinaigrette, which pairs beautifully with classic Mediterranean ingredients like marinated artichoke hearts and sun-dried tomatoes. It's fiber-rich thanks to the addition of cannellini beans and loaded with protein-packed tuna. It's definitely a departure from the salad of your childhood. Who knew being a grown-up could taste so good?

SERVINGS: **1**   PREP TIME: **5 MINUTES**

---

1 (5-ounce) can tuna, drained and flaked

½ cup canned cannellini beans, drained and rinsed

¼ cup chopped marinated artichoke hearts

¼ cup chopped sun-dried tomatoes

¼ cup chopped pitted Kalamata olives

2 tablespoons Italian Dressing (page 226)

2 cups baby spinach (3 to 4 ounces)

IN a bowl, combine the tuna, cannellini beans, artichoke hearts, sun-dried tomatoes, olives, and dressing. Toss gently until everything is evenly dressed.

SERVE the tuna mixture on a plate over a bed of baby spinach or store in the refrigerator for up to 3 days.

simple swaps

If you're not a fan of tuna, swap in 5 ounces shredded cooked chicken.

mix it up

For a more filling lunch, try replacing 1 cup of the baby spinach with 1 cup cooked rice or quinoa (see page 34).

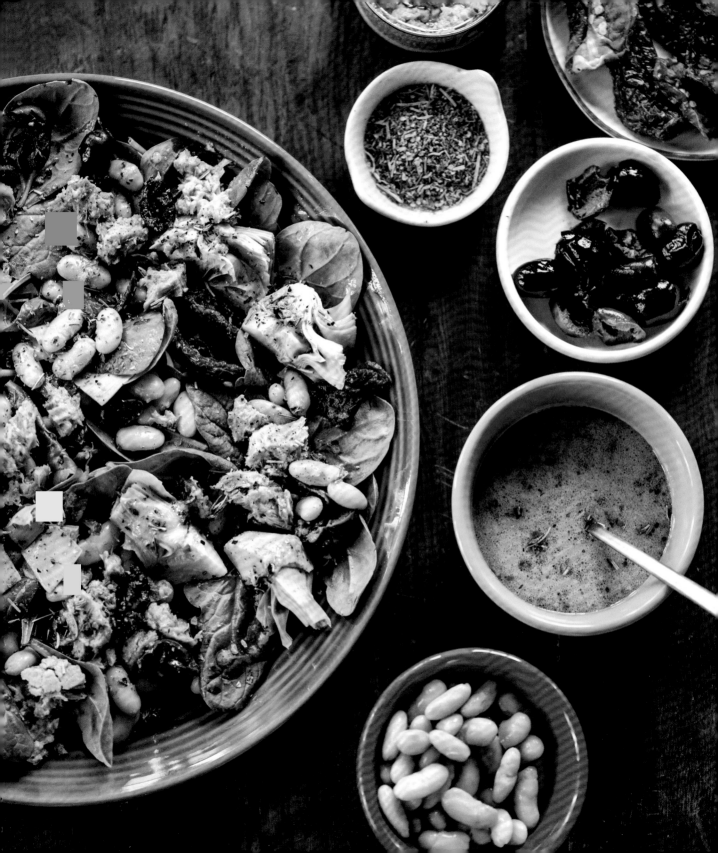

FRESH RAINBOW ROLLS WITH TANGY PEANUT SAUCE

You're probably familiar with the concept of "Eat the Rainbow." The idea is basically that if you're eating lots of bright, colorful fruits and veggies, you're more likely to be getting a good array of nutrients in your diet. That's the inspiration behind these incredibly tasty and incredibly vibrant Fresh Rainbow Rolls. And while they do take a little time to prepare, I promise it will be love at first bite.

SERVINGS: **4**   PREP TIME: **30 MINUTES**

¾ cup smooth natural peanut butter

¼ cup fresh lime juice

3 tablespoons soy sauce

2 tablespoons coconut sugar

1 tablespoon sriracha sauce (optional)

1 teaspoon grated fresh ginger

Hot water, as needed

1 cup cooked rice vermicelli noodles

½ English cucumber, julienned

½ cup shredded red cabbage

1 mango, julienned

2 carrots, julienned

1 red bell pepper, thinly sliced

4 green onions, thinly sliced

¼ cup fresh cilantro leaves

20 round rice paper wrappers

IN a bowl, whisk together the peanut butter, lime juice, soy sauce, coconut sugar, sriracha (if using), and ginger. Gradually whisk in hot water as needed to thin the dip to the desired consistency.

HAVE the fruit and vegetables prepped and laid out on a plate so they're easy to access.

SOAK one rice paper round in warm water for 15 seconds and then lay it flat on a cutting board. In the center of the lower third of the round, arrange a few slices of each fruit and vegetable and top with some noodles. Finish with the cilantro. Wrap the ingredients in the rice paper like a burrito: Start by wrapping the bottom of the rice paper over the filling and tucking in the filling as you roll. About halfway up, fold the sides of the rice paper in toward the center and continue rolling. Set aside on a plate and cover lightly with a damp paper towel. Repeat with the remaining ingredients.

ENJOY immediately, with the sauce alongside for dipping, or store in an airtight container with a wet paper towel (to keep them moist) in the refrigerator for up to 3 days. I recommend replacing the paper towel each day.

simple swaps

You can switch up the dip by replacing the Tangy Peanut Sauce with some sweet Thai chili sauce.

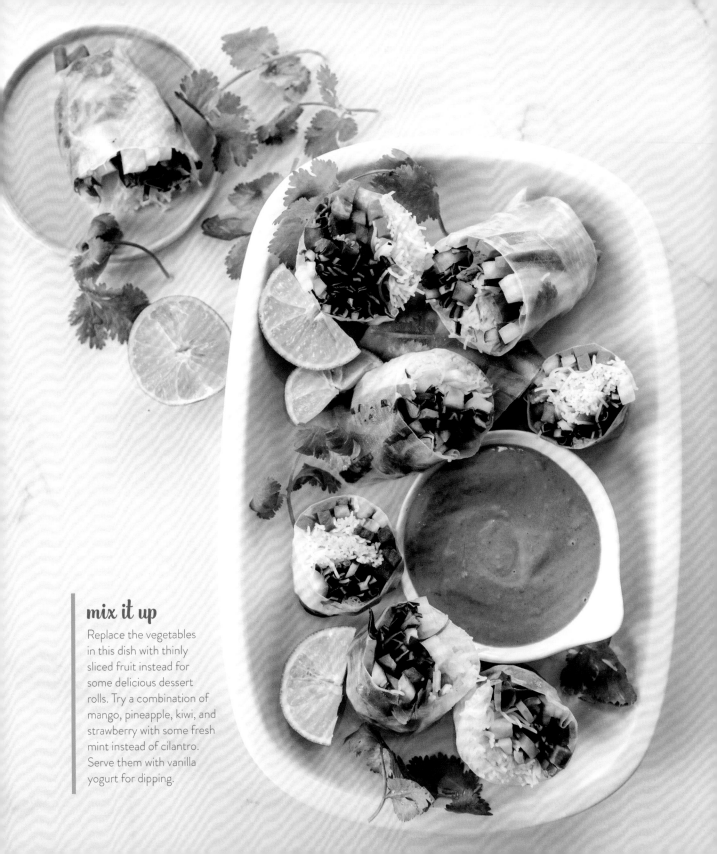

mix it up

Replace the vegetables in this dish with thinly sliced fruit instead for some delicious dessert rolls. Try a combination of mango, pineapple, kiwi, and strawberry with some fresh mint instead of cilantro. Serve them with vanilla yogurt for dipping.

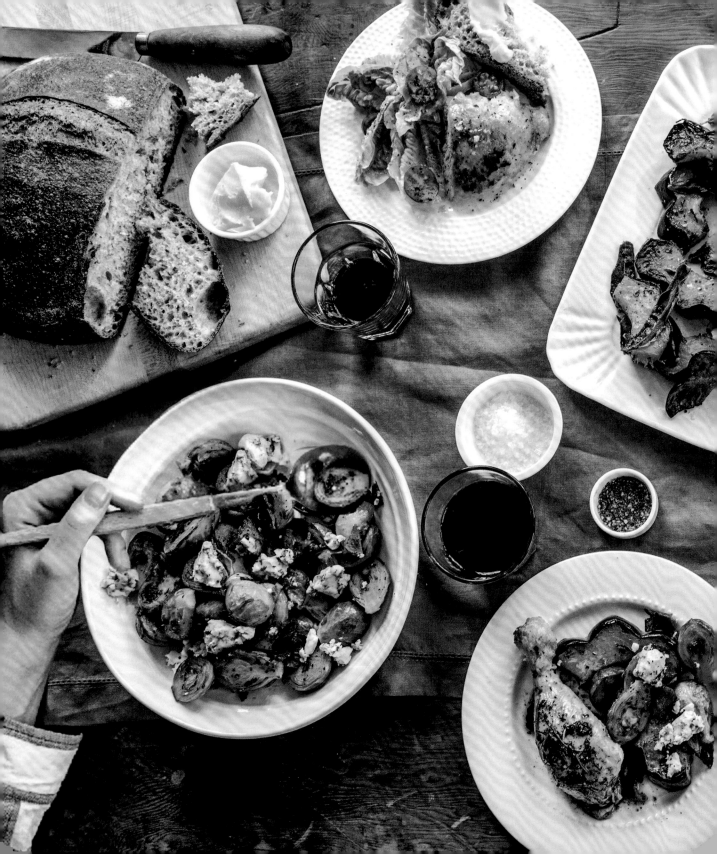

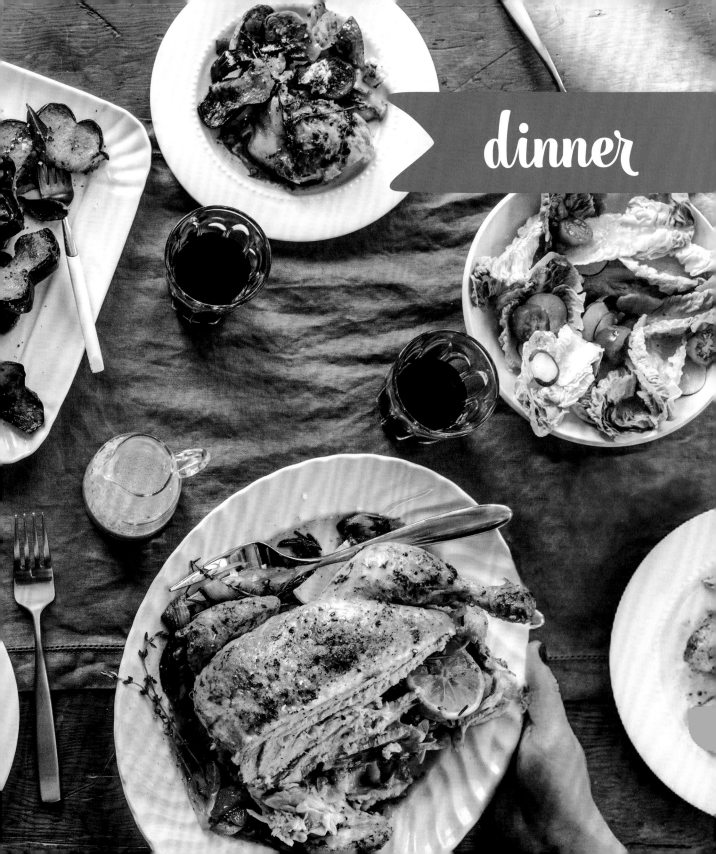

dinner

TURKEY TACO QUINOA SKILLET

Skillet suppers have long been my go-to for easy weeknight cooking—they're fast and convenient, and above all, they make cleanup a breeze. But don't mistake effortless for flavorless; this Turkey Taco Quinoa Skillet is bursting with zesty Southwestern flavors that are sure to satisfy. It's also loaded with protein and lots of veggies. This dish is a perfect make-ahead meal, so make a double batch and enjoy it for lunch or freeze the leftovers.

SERVINGS: **6** PREP TIME: **10 MINUTES** COOK TIME: **30 TO 35 MINUTES**

1 tablespoon vegetable oil

1 small yellow onion, diced

1 red bell pepper, diced

1 pound ground turkey

2 garlic cloves, minced

½ jalapeño, minced

1 tablespoon chili powder

1 teaspoon ground cumin

2½ cups chicken broth, homemade (page 206) or store-bought

1 (15-ounce) can black beans, drained and rinsed

1 (14.5-ounce) can diced tomatoes

1 cup fresh or frozen corn kernels

1 cup quinoa

Juice of 1 lime

1 tablespoon chopped fresh cilantro

Salt and freshly ground black pepper

½ cup grated cheddar cheese

Sour cream, for serving

IN a large skillet with a lid, heat the vegetable oil over medium-high heat. Add the onion and bell pepper and cook, stirring, until they begin to soften, 3 to 4 minutes. Add the ground turkey and cook, breaking it up with a spoon as it cooks, until browned, about 6 minutes. Stir in the garlic, jalapeño, chili powder, and cumin and cook, stirring, until they become fragrant, about 30 seconds. Add the broth, black beans, tomatoes, corn, and quinoa and bring the mixture to a simmer.

REDUCE the heat to medium-low, cover, and cook until the quinoa is cooked through and most of the liquid has been absorbed, about 20 minutes.

STIR in the lime juice and cilantro and season with salt and pepper. Top evenly with the cheese, cover the skillet, and allow the cheese to melt, 1 to 2 minutes.

SERVE immediately, with a dollop of sour cream, or store in the refrigerator for up to 3 days.

(continued)

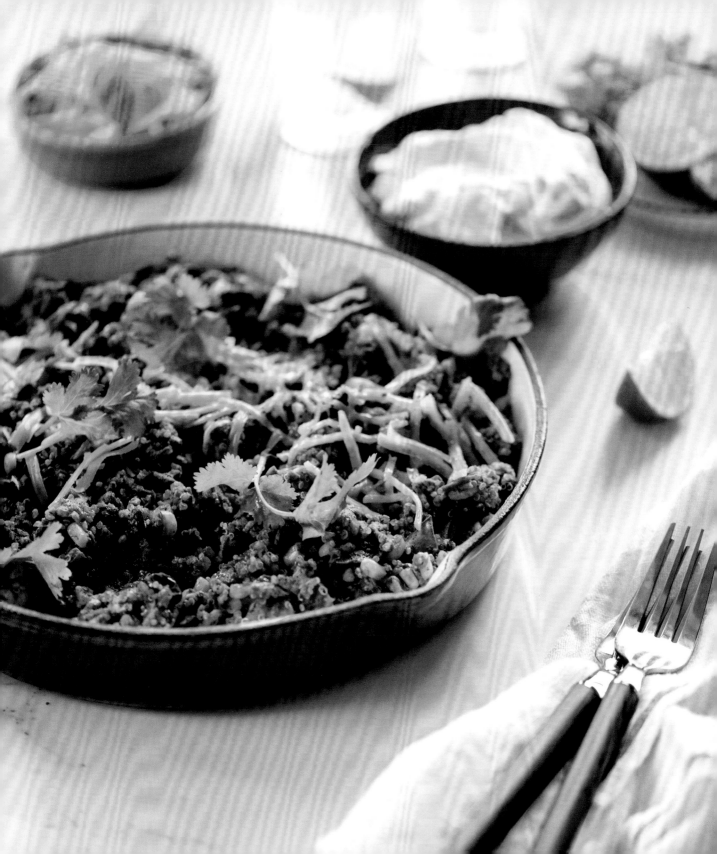

(Turkey Taco Quinoa Skillet continued)

mix it up

Try adding 1 minced chipotle pepper in adobo sauce for some smokiness, or if you're looking for a bit of a kick, finish each serving with 1 tablespoon Salsa Verde (page 215).

simple swaps

- Feel free to swap out the ground turkey for beef, chicken, or veggie crumbles—they all work great!
- If you're not a fan of quinoa, use rice instead and cook for as long as the package directions indicate.
- The cheddar cheese is completely optional, so if you'd like to keep this dish dairy-free, just leave it out.

HEALTHY CHICKEN PICCATA

WHEAT-FREE

DAIRY-FREE

This Healthy Chicken Piccata is filled with flavor thanks to high-impact ingredients like garlic, lemon, and capers. In my lightened-up version of this classic Italian dish, I've skipped the traditional breading altogether and kept it completely gluten-free. But what I love most about it is how quickly it comes together—and all in a single pan! Pure weeknight perfection.

SERVINGS: **4**   PREP TIME: **5 MINUTES**   COOK TIME: **30 MINUTES**

---

4 boneless, skinless chicken breasts

Salt and freshly ground black pepper

2 tablespoons extra-virgin olive oil

2 tablespoons capers

2 garlic cloves, minced

1 cup chicken broth, homemade (page 206) or store-bought

½ cup white wine

Grated zest and juice of 1 lemon

1 tablespoon cornstarch

2 tablespoons water

2 tablespoons chopped fresh parsley

SEASON the chicken breasts generously on both sides with salt and pepper.

IN a large skillet with a lid, heat 1 tablespoon of the olive oil over medium-high heat. Add the chicken breasts and cook until they are nicely browned on the first side and release easily from the pan, about 6 minutes. Flip the chicken and cook on the second side for 4 minutes. Transfer the chicken to a plate.

IN the same skillet, heat the remaining 1 tablespoon olive oil. Add the capers and garlic and cook until fragrant, about 30 seconds. Add the broth, wine, lemon zest, and lemon juice. Bring the mixture to a boil and return the chicken to the pan. Reduce the heat to medium-low, cover, and simmer for 15 minutes, or until a meat thermometer inserted into each chicken breast registers 165°F. Remove the chicken from the pan and set aside on a large plate.

IN a small bowl, whisk together the cornstarch and water until the cornstarch has dissolved. Stir the cornstarch slurry into the juices in the pan and simmer for 1 to 2 minutes more, until thickened slightly. Stir in the parsley.

SERVE the chicken topped with the pan sauce. Leftovers can be stored in the refrigerator for up to 3 days.

mix it up

While chicken piccata is a classic, firm white-fleshed fish like cod or tilapia can be used in this recipe instead. Cooking times will need to be adjusted slightly, since fish cooks fairly quickly, but the results will be equally delicious.

BETTER-THAN-TAKEOUT ORANGE CHICKEN

DAIRY-FREE

Trust me, I totally understand how tempting take-out can be on a weeknight when you just don't feel like cooking, but you might be surprised how simple it can be to prepare your very own version at home. This easy Orange Chicken is exceptionally flavorful but boasts a lot less sodium and far fewer calories than its restaurant counterpart. I like to serve this dish over cooked rice or quinoa with a side of my delicious Chili-Garlic Broccoli (page 182).

SERVINGS: **4**   PREP TIME: **10 MINUTES**   COOK TIME: **15 MINUTES**

Grated zest and juice of 1 large navel orange

3 tablespoons soy sauce

2 tablespoons honey

2 tablespoons cornstarch

1 garlic clove, minced

½ teaspoon grated fresh ginger

1 tablespoon vegetable oil

2 boneless, skinless chicken breasts, cut into 1-inch cubes

1 red bell pepper, thinly sliced

2 cups snap peas, strings removed

2 green onions, thinly sliced

1 teaspoon sesame seeds

IN a small bowl, whisk together the orange zest, orange juice, soy sauce, honey, cornstarch, garlic, and ginger until well combined.

IN a large wok or nonstick skillet, heat the vegetable oil over medium-high heat. Add the chicken and cook, stirring often, until it is golden on the outside and no longer pink inside, 6 to 8 minutes. Add the bell pepper and cook, stirring, for 2 minutes. Add the orange sauce and snap peas and cook, stirring, until the sauce has thickened and the peas are tender-crisp, 3 to 4 minutes.

GARNISH with the green onions and sesame seeds.

SERVE immediately or store in the refrigerator for up to 3 days.

simple swaps

You can easily replace the chicken in this recipe with 8 ounces extra-firm tofu, cut into ¾-inch cubes. Simply toss the tofu in 2 tablespoons cornstarch before adding it to the pan to get a nice, crisp exterior. Cook the tofu in the vegetable oil, stirring often, until it becomes golden, about 6 minutes.

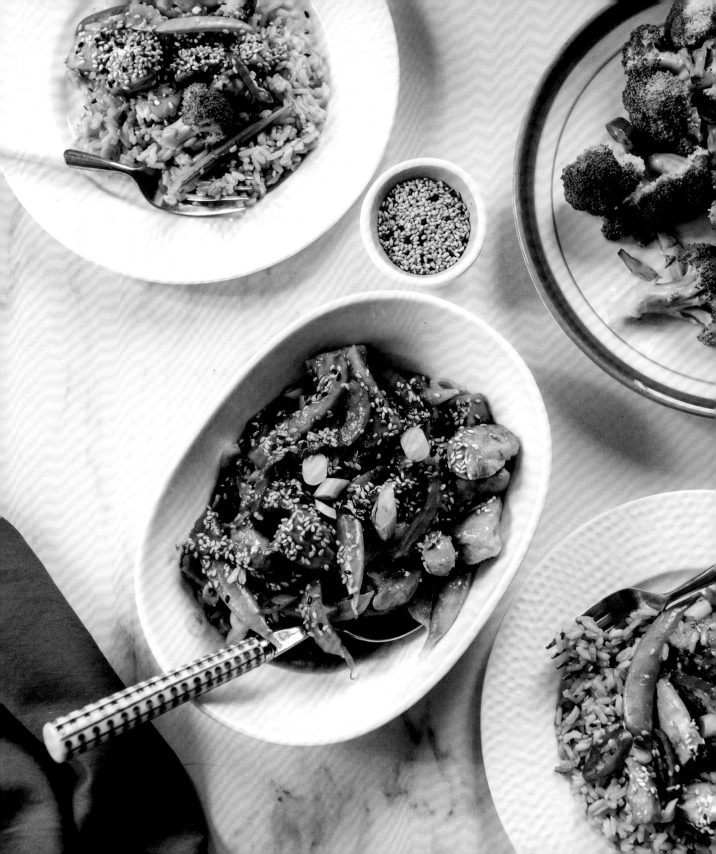

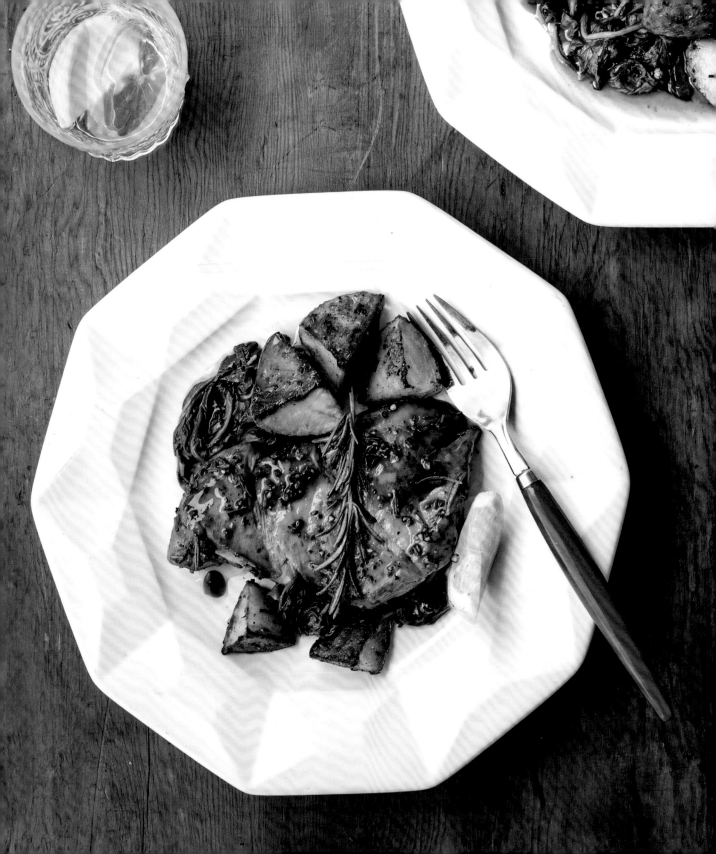

BALSAMIC-GLAZED CHICKEN

WHEAT-FREE
DAIRY-FREE

While we know they're an exceptional source of lean protein, boneless, skinless chicken breasts are notoriously bland, so getting people excited to eat them is no small feat. That's why my Balsamic-Glazed Chicken is such a game changer. It's the perfect balance of sweet, savory, and a little tart (thanks to the balsamic vinegar), so what you end up with is a healthy chicken dish that doesn't disappoint. And you'll want to be sure to make a little extra, since this recipe is perfect for lunch as well.

SERVINGS: **4**   PREP TIME: **5 MINUTES**   COOK TIME: **20 MINUTES**

½ cup chicken broth, homemade (page 206) or store-bought

3 tablespoons balsamic vinegar

2 tablespoons honey

1 tablespoon finely chopped fresh rosemary, plus a few sprigs for garnish

4 boneless, skinless chicken breasts

Salt and freshly ground black pepper

2 tablespoons vegetable oil

IN a small bowl, whisk together the broth, vinegar, honey, and rosemary until well combined.

SEASON the chicken breasts generously with salt and pepper. In a large skillet with a lid, heat the vegetable oil over medium-high heat. Arrange the chicken breasts in the skillet, rounded-side down, and cook, undisturbed, until the chicken is golden brown on the first side and releases easily from the pan, 4 to 6 minutes. Use tongs to flip the chicken and cook on the second side for 3 to 4 minutes.

POUR the vinegar mixture over the chicken. Reduce the heat to medium-low and cook, flipping the chicken every few minutes, until the glaze has reduced and a meat thermometer inserted into the thickest part of each chicken breast registers 165°F, about 10 minutes.

SERVE the chicken immediately, with a drizzle of glaze from the pan and a sprig of rosemary, or store in the refrigerator for up to 3 days.

simple swaps

For a more affordable (and I think more flavorful) dish, try using bone-in, skin-on chicken legs instead of breasts.

mix it up

This same tasty glaze is delicious with potatoes. Preheat the oven to 375°F. Cut some well-washed red potatoes into wedges, put them in a large bowl, and pour over the glaze. Season with salt and pepper, transfer to a baking sheet, and roast, tossing the potatoes regularly, until tender, about 30 minutes.

DINNER

BAKED SALMON

When you're talking about meals made *easy*, Baked Salmon simply can't be overlooked. In addition to being loaded with protein and heart-healthy omega-3s, it's effortless to prepare, making it a must for your weeknight dinner rotation. And if you can spare an hour to let it soak in a tasty marinade, your patience will most certainly be rewarded by the flavor gods. Here are three of my fave ways to enjoy it . . .

CLASSIC LEMON & DILL SALMON

SERVINGS: **4**   PREP TIME: **1 HOUR 5 MINUTES**   COOK TIME: **15 MINUTES**

WHEAT-FREE
DAIRY-FREE
PESCATARIAN

¼ cup extra-virgin olive oil

Grated zest and juice of 1 lemon, plus 4 lemon slices for serving

2 garlic cloves, minced

¼ cup chopped fresh dill

4 (4-ounce) salmon fillets

Salt and freshly ground black pepper

IN a small bowl, whisk together the olive oil, lemon zest, lemon juice, garlic, and dill until well combined.

PLACE the salmon fillets in a large zipper bag. Pour the marinade over the salmon. Close the bag and massage the fillets until they are evenly coated in the marinade. Refrigerate for at least 1 hour or up to overnight.

WHEN it's time to cook the salmon, preheat the oven to 450°F. Line a baking sheet with parchment paper.

ARRANGE the fillets skin-side down on the prepared baking sheet. Be sure to discard any remaining marinade. Season each fillet with salt and pepper. Place a lemon slice on each.

BAKE for 12 to 15 minutes, until the salmon is firm and flakes easily with a fork.

SERVE immediately or store in the refrigerator for up to 3 days.

simple swaps

You can replace the dill in this recipe with 2 tablespoons chopped fresh tarragon.

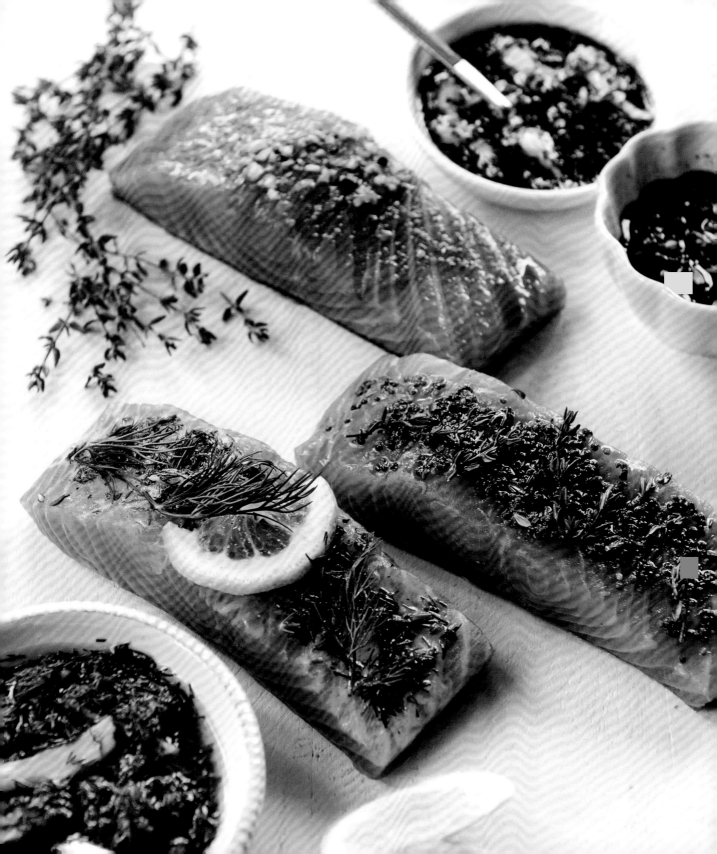

MAPLE-DIJON SALMON

SERVINGS: **4**   PREP TIME: **1 HOUR 5 MINUTES**   COOK TIME: **15 MINUTES**

WHEAT-FREE
DAIRY-FREE
PESCATARIAN

¼ cup maple syrup

2 tablespoons grainy Dijon mustard

2 garlic cloves, minced

1 teaspoon fresh thyme leaves

4 (4-ounce) salmon fillets

Salt and freshly ground black pepper

IN a small bowl, whisk together the maple syrup, mustard, garlic, and thyme until well combined.

PLACE the salmon fillets in a large zipper bag. Pour the marinade over the salmon. Close the bag and massage the fillets until they are evenly coated in the marinade. Refrigerate for at least 1 hour or up to overnight.

WHEN it's time to cook the salmon, preheat the oven to 450°F. Line a baking sheet with parchment paper.

ARRANGE the fillets skin-side down on the prepared baking sheet. Be sure to discard the remaining marinade. Season each fillet with salt and pepper.

BAKE for 12 to 15 minutes, until the salmon is firm and flakes easily with a fork.

SERVE immediately or store in the refrigerator for up to 3 days.

mix it up

This wonderful sweet-and-savory marinade is also amazing on pork chops.

SWEET & SPICY SRIRACHA SALMON

DAIRY-FREE

PESCATARIAN

SERVINGS: **4**   PREP TIME: **1 HOUR 5 MINUTES**   COOK TIME: **15 MINUTES**

¼ cup soy sauce

2 tablespoons honey

1 tablespoon sriracha sauce

1 tablespoon rice vinegar

2 teaspoons grated fresh ginger

2 garlic cloves, minced

4 (4-ounce) salmon fillets

Chopped green onions, for serving

IN a small bowl, whisk together the soy sauce, honey, sriracha, vinegar, ginger, and garlic until well combined.

PLACE the salmon fillets in a large zipper bag. Pour the marinade over the salmon. Close the bag and massage the fillets until they are evenly coated in the marinade. Refrigerate for at least 1 hour or up to overnight.

WHEN it's time to cook the salmon, preheat the oven to 450°F. Line a baking sheet with parchment paper.

ARRANGE the fillets skin-side down on the prepared baking sheet. Be sure to discard the remaining marinade.

BAKE for 12 to 15 minutes, until the salmon is firm and flakes easily with a fork.

SERVE immediately, garnished with green onions, or store in the refrigerator for up to 3 days.

simple swaps

If you're looking for a gluten-free alternative to soy sauce, use gluten-free tamari instead.

STEAK SALAD WITH WARM TOMATO VINAIGRETTE

It's not often that I find a salad hearty enough to reach supper-worthy status, but this one does just that. The flavorful combination of juicy medium-rare steak, peppery arugula, tart tomato vinaigrette, and pungent blue cheese just might be one of the best things you eat this year. This dish is perfect during the summer months when the grill is fired up, but you can also enjoy it off-season by simply cooking your steak on the stovetop in a cast-iron skillet instead.

SERVINGS: **2**   PREP TIME: **10 MINUTES**   COOK TIME: **15 MINUTES**

---

1 (8-ounce) New York strip steak

1½ tablespoons extra-virgin olive oil

Salt and freshly ground black pepper

1 shallot, minced

1 garlic clove, minced

1 cup halved cherry tomatoes

2 tablespoons red wine vinegar

2 tablespoons chopped fresh basil

6 cups arugula

⅓ cup crumbled blue cheese

HEAT a grill to high.

BRUSH the steak with 1½ teaspoons of the olive oil and season it liberally on both sides with salt and pepper.

PLACE the steak on the hot grill and cook until golden brown and lightly charred on the first side, about 4 minutes. Flip the steak and cook until grill marks develop on the second side, 3 to 4 minutes, or to your desired doneness; for medium-rare, cook until a meat thermometer registers 135°F. Transfer the steak to a cutting board. Let rest for 5 minutes before slicing the steak into ¼-inch-thick strips.

IN the meantime, in a medium skillet, heat the remaining 1 tablespoon olive oil over medium-high heat. Add the shallot and cook, stirring, until it begins to soften, about 2 minutes. Stir in the garlic and cook until fragrant, about 30 seconds. Add the tomatoes and vinegar and cook, stirring, until the tomatoes soften and begin to release their juices, about 3 minutes. Turn off the heat, stir in the basil, and season with salt and pepper.

PUT the arugula in a large serving bowl and place the steak slices on top. Pour over the warm tomato vinaigrette and finish with the blue cheese.

SERVE immediately.

mix it up

If you don't eat red meat, you can always swap out the steak for some grilled chicken breast or skip the meat entirely to make this dish completely vegetarian.

CHIPOTLE CHICKEN CHILI

WHEAT-FREE

This hearty but healthy Chipotle Chicken Chili is the perfect dish to cozy up to on a cold day. It's wonderfully smoky, just a little spicy, and deeply satisfying, which makes it totally worth the time it takes to prepare. It's one of my very favorite ways to use leftover chicken, and it's also a great place to hide extra veggies when no one is looking—bonus!

SERVINGS: **6**   PREP TIME: **15 MINUTES**   COOK TIME: **40 MINUTES**

---

2 tablespoons vegetable oil

1 small yellow onion, diced

2 celery stalks, diced

1 red bell pepper, diced

3 garlic cloves, minced

1 or 2 canned chipotle peppers in adobo sauce, minced

2 tablespoons chili powder

1 tablespoon ground cumin

1 tablespoon garlic powder

1 teaspoon dried oregano

2 cups shredded cooked chicken breast

2 (15-ounce) cans black beans, drained and rinsed

1 (28-ounce) can diced tomatoes

1 (28-ounce) can crushed tomatoes

2 cups chicken broth, homemade (page 206) or store-bought

1 cup fresh or frozen corn kernels

Salt and freshly ground black pepper

½ cup sour cream, for serving

½ cup shredded sharp cheddar cheese, for serving

2 green onions, thinly sliced, for serving

IN a large soup pot or Dutch oven, heat the vegetable oil over medium-high heat. Add the onion, celery, and bell pepper and cook, stirring, until softened, about 5 minutes. Stir in the garlic and cook for another minute. Add the chipotle peppers, chili powder, cumin, garlic powder, and oregano. Cook for another minute to really bring out the flavors of the spices.

ADD the chicken, black beans, diced tomatoes, crushed tomatoes, broth, and corn and stir well. Bring to a boil, then cover and reduce the heat to medium-low. Simmer the chili, stirring occasionally, for at least 30 minutes or up to 2 hours to develop the best flavor. Season with salt and pepper.

(continued)

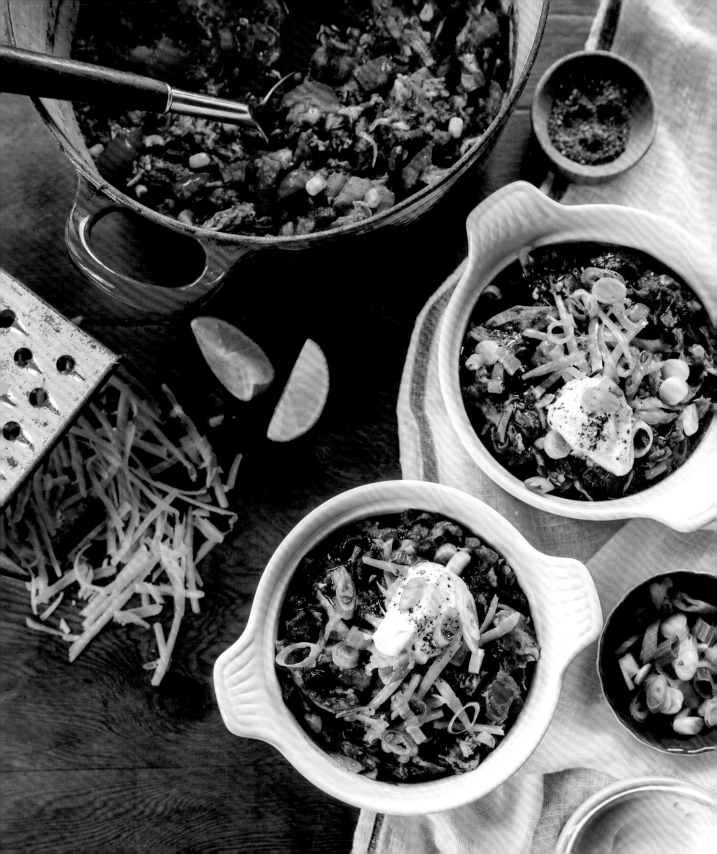

(Chipotle Chicken Chili continued)

SERVE hot, topped with the sour cream, cheddar cheese, and green onions, or let cool and store in the refrigerator for up to 3 days or in the freezer for up to 3 months. Reheat and top with the sour cream, cheese, and green onions just before serving.

simple swaps

The black beans in this recipe can easily be replaced with canned red kidney beans or even chickpeas.

mix it up

For a vegetarian version of this delicious chili, simply swap out the cooked chicken for veggie crumbles and the chicken broth for vegetable broth. It's one of my favorite dishes for Meatless Monday.

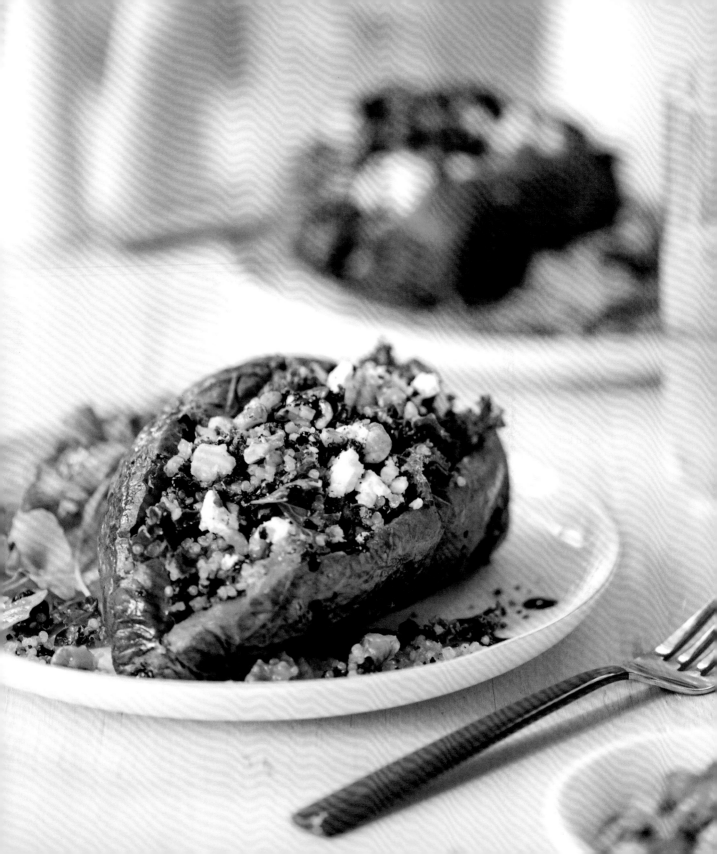

STUFFED SWEET POTATOES

Stuffed Sweet Potatoes make a healthy and filling weeknight dinner. To give yourself an edge, bake your sweet potatoes during your Sunday meal prep and store them in the refrigerator until you're ready to use them. They can be reheated quickly in the microwave or in the oven and then stuffed with all sorts of deliciousness . . .

KALE & QUINOA STUFFED SWEET POTATOES

VEGETARIAN
WHEAT-FREE
PESCATARIAN

SERVINGS: **2**   PREP TIME: **10 MINUTES**   COOK TIME: **1 HOUR 5 MINUTES**

2 large sweet potatoes

1 teaspoon vegetable oil

¼ teaspoon salt

1 cup chopped kale leaves

1 teaspoon extra-virgin olive oil

1 cup cooked quinoa (see page 34)

¼ cup crumbled goat cheese

¼ cup dried cranberries

¼ cup chopped walnuts

2 teaspoons honey

PREHEAT the oven to 400°F. Line a baking sheet with parchment paper or aluminum foil.

SCRUB the sweet potatoes thoroughly using a vegetable brush. Pat them dry with a kitchen towel. Using a fork, carefully pierce the top of the sweet potatoes four or five times. Rub the skin with the vegetable oil and season with the salt. Place the sweet potatoes on the prepared baking sheet and bake for about 1 hour, or until they are fork-tender. Remove from the oven (keep the oven on) and set aside until just cool enough to handle.

WHILE the sweet potatoes bake, put the kale in a large bowl and add the olive oil. Using clean hands, massage the oil into the kale until the leaves are tender, about 2 minutes.

CUT the sweet potatoes in half lengthwise and, using a fork, fluff the flesh of the potato halves. Top each of the halves evenly with the quinoa, kale, goat cheese, dried cranberries, and walnuts. Bake for 5 minutes more.

DRIZZLE evenly with the honey and serve immediately or store in the refrigerator for up to 3 days.

ROAST TURKEY STUFFED SWEET POTATOES

WHEAT-FREE

DAIRY-FREE

SERVINGS: **2**   PREP TIME: **5 MINUTES**   COOK TIME: **1 HOUR 5 MINUTES**

2 large sweet potatoes

1 teaspoon vegetable oil

¼ teaspoon salt, plus more as needed

2 cups shredded roast turkey

½ cup cranberry sauce

¼ cup chopped pecans

½ teaspoon fresh thyme leaves

Freshly ground black pepper

PREHEAT the oven to 400°F. Line a baking sheet with parchment paper or aluminum foil.

SCRUB the sweet potatoes thoroughly using a vegetable brush. Pat them dry with a kitchen towel. Using a fork, carefully pierce the top of the sweet potatoes four or five times. Rub the skin with the vegetable oil and season with the salt. Place the sweet potatoes on the prepared baking sheet and bake for about 1 hour, or until they are fork-tender. Remove from the oven (keep the oven on) and set aside until just cool enough to handle.

CUT the sweet potatoes in half lengthwise and, using a fork, fluff the flesh of the potato halves. Top each half evenly with the roast turkey, cranberry sauce, pecans, and thyme. Season with salt and pepper and bake for 5 minutes more.

SERVE immediately or store in the refrigerator for up to 3 days.

simple swaps

This is a great way to use turkey leftovers after the holidays, but if you don't have any on hand, simply swap in some oven-roasted turkey slices from the deli.

SOUTHWESTERN STUFFED SWEET POTATOES

VEGETARIAN
WHEAT-FREE
PESCATARIAN

SERVINGS: **2**   PREP TIME: **5 MINUTES**   COOK TIME: **1 HOUR 5 MINUTES**

2 large sweet potatoes

1 teaspoon vegetable oil

¼ teaspoon salt, plus more as needed

1 cup black beans, drained and rinsed

½ cup fresh or frozen corn kernels

¼ cup salsa fresca, homemade (page 214) or store-bought

½ teaspoon chili powder

Grated zest and juice of 1 lime

¼ cup shredded cheddar cheese

Fresh cilantro, for garnish

PREHEAT the oven to 400°F. Line a baking sheet with parchment paper or aluminum foil.

SCRUB the sweet potatoes thoroughly using a vegetable brush. Pat them dry with a kitchen towel. Using a fork, carefully pierce the top of the sweet potatoes four or five times. Rub the skin with the vegetable oil and season with the salt. Place the sweet potatoes on the prepared baking sheet and bake for about 1 hour, or until they are fork-tender. Remove from the oven (keep the oven on) and set aside until just cool enough to handle.

CUT the sweet potatoes in half lengthwise and, using a fork, fluff the flesh of the potato halves.

IN a medium bowl, combine the black beans, corn, salsa, chili powder, lime zest, and lime juice. Toss well. Divide the mixture evenly between the sweet potato halves. Top each with half the cheese and bake for 5 minutes more.

SERVE immediately, garnished with fresh cilantro, or store in the refrigerator for up to 3 days.

SHEET PAN SUPPERS

As you may have guessed by now, "easy" is my mantra in the kitchen, and Sheet Pan Suppers are about as easy as it gets. Each of these nutritious, protein-packed dinner recipes can be prepared effortlessly using just a single baking sheet.

HALIBUT WITH GREEN BEANS, TOMATOES & OLIVES

WHEAT-FREE
DAIRY-FREE
PESCATARIAN

SERVINGS: **4**   PREP TIME: **5 MINUTES**   COOK TIME: **35 MINUTES**

3 cups halved baby potatoes

2 tablespoons extra-virgin olive oil

½ teaspoon garlic powder

Salt and freshly ground black pepper

½ pound green beans, trimmed

1 cup cherry tomatoes

½ cup pitted Kalamata olives

2 tablespoons capers

4 (4-ounce) halibut fillets

PREHEAT the oven to 400°F.

IN a large bowl, toss the potatoes with 1 tablespoon of the olive oil, the garlic powder, and salt and pepper.

TRANSFER the potatoes to a baking sheet, spread them in an even layer, and bake for about 20 minutes, or until they begin to brown.

REMOVE the potatoes from the oven and toss them gently. Add the green beans, tomatoes, olives, and capers to the baking sheet. Arrange the halibut fillets in the center of the pan. Drizzle everything with the remaining 1 tablespoon olive oil and season with salt and pepper.

BAKE until the halibut fillets are cooked through and flake easily with a fork, about 15 minutes.

SERVE immediately or let cool completely and store in the refrigerator for up to 3 days.

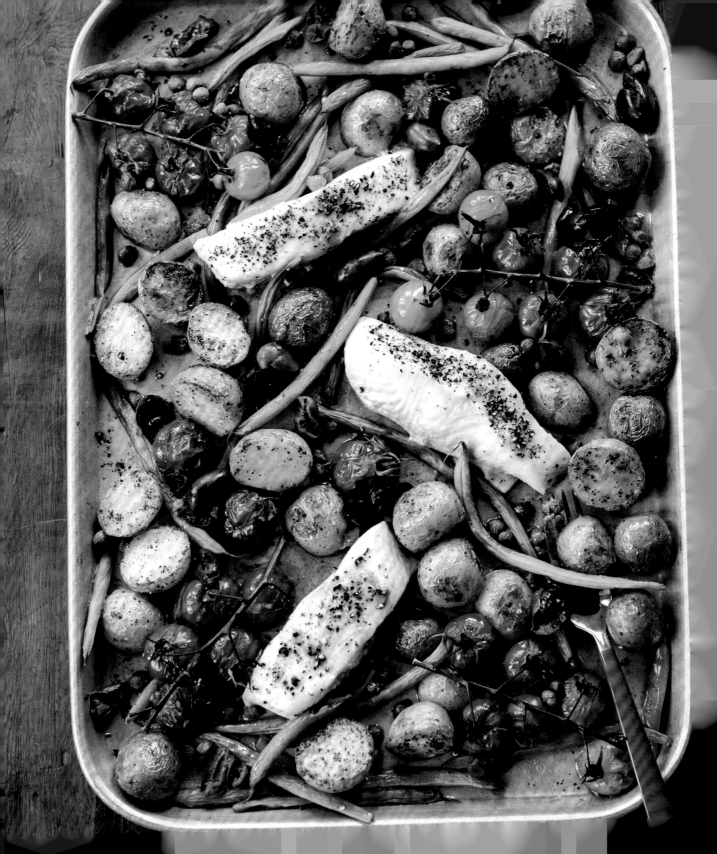

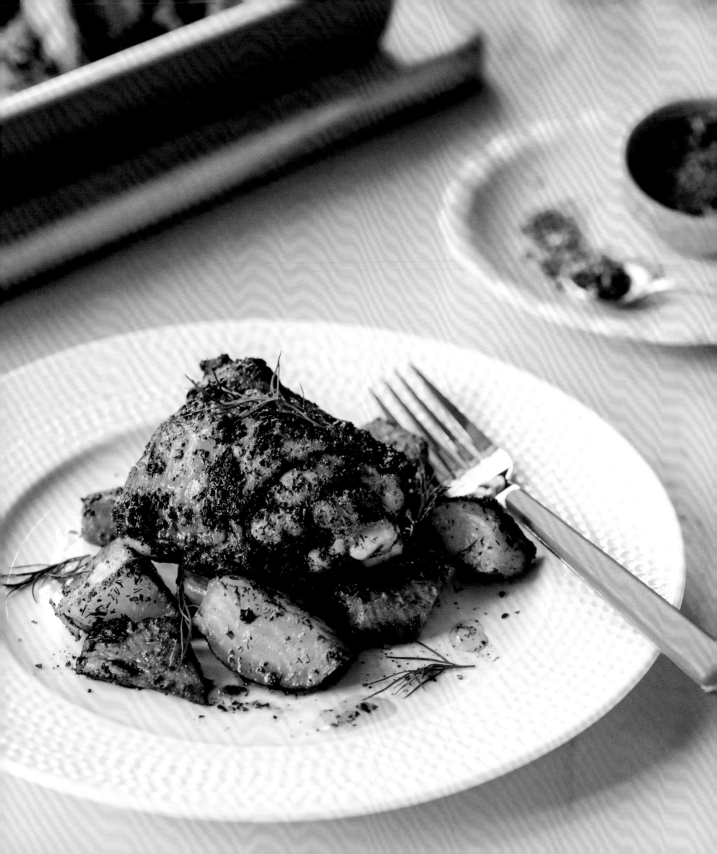

RANCH ROASTED CHICKEN & VEGGIES

WHEAT-FREE
DAIRY-FREE

SERVINGS: **4**   PREP TIME: **5 MINUTES**   COOK TIME: **50 MINUTES**

4 chicken legs, separated into drumsticks and thighs

4 red potatoes, washed and cubed

4 medium carrots, chopped

2 tablespoons extra-virgin olive oil

2 tablespoons Ranch Seasoning (page 231)

Salt and freshly ground black pepper

Fresh dill, for garnish

PREHEAT the oven to 375°F.

ARRANGE the chicken, potatoes, and carrots on a large baking sheet. Drizzle with the olive oil and season liberally with the Ranch Seasoning and salt and pepper.

BAKE until the vegetables are tender and the chicken is golden brown, about 45 minutes. The chicken should read 165°F on a meat thermometer. Switch the oven to the broil setting and broil until the chicken skin is crisp and golden, about 4 minutes.

SERVE immediately, garnished with fresh dill, or let cool completely and store in the refrigerator for up to 3 days.

DINNER

CHILI-LIME SHRIMP FAJITAS

SERVINGS: **4**   PREP TIME: **10 MINUTES**   COOK TIME: **10 MINUTES**

1 red bell pepper, thinly sliced

1 orange bell pepper, thinly sliced

1 small red onion, thinly sliced

½ jalapeño, thinly sliced (optional)

1 pound large shrimp, peeled and deveined

2 tablespoons extra-virgin olive oil

1 tablespoon chili powder

½ teaspoon garlic powder

Salt and freshly ground black pepper

Grated zest and juice of 1 lime

4 to 6 large corn tortillas

½ cup Guacamole (page 218), for serving

¼ cup sour cream, for serving

Fresh cilantro, for serving

PREHEAT the oven to 400°F.

IN a large bowl, combine the bell peppers, onion, jalapeño (if using), shrimp, olive oil, chili powder, garlic powder, and salt and pepper. Toss with tongs until all the ingredients are well coated.

ARRANGE the mixture in an even layer on a baking sheet. Bake for 10 minutes, until the shrimp are pink and opaque and the vegetables have softened. Remove the pan from the oven. Sprinkle with the lime zest and juice and toss to coat.

SERVE immediately, with the tortillas, guacamole, sour cream, and cilantro, or let cool completely and store in the refrigerator for up to 3 days.

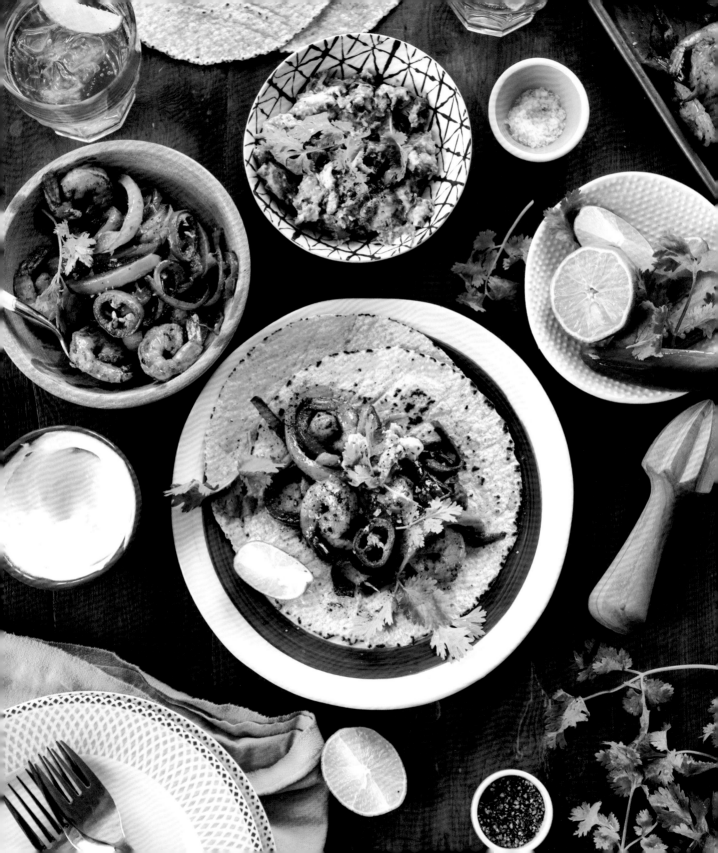

FALAFEL BURGER

These delicious vegetarian burgers are the perfect way to celebrate the arrival of summer. They're fresh tasting, full of good-for-you ingredients, and—best of all—they can be made in advance, so they're perfect for entertaining. If the weather isn't quite cooperative enough for BBQing, cook these inside on a skillet. Either way, you'll be glad you did!

SERVINGS: **4**   PREP TIME: **25 MINUTES**   COOK TIME: **8 MINUTES**

2 (15-ounce) cans chickpeas, drained and rinsed

½ cup bread crumbs

½ small red onion, chopped

¼ cup chopped fresh parsley

1 large egg

2 garlic cloves, minced

Grated zest and juice of 1 lemon

1 teaspoon ground cumin

½ teaspoon ground coriander

Salt and freshly ground black pepper

1 tablespoon extra-virgin olive oil

4 hamburger buns

1 medium tomato, cut into 4 slices

4 Bibb lettuce leaves

¼ cup Tzatziki Sauce (page 222)

IN a food processor, combine the chickpeas, bread crumbs, red onion, parsley, egg, garlic, lemon zest, lemon juice, cumin, and coriander. Season with salt and pepper. Slowly pulse until the ingredients are well incorporated and the mixture resembles coarse crumbs. Do not overmix—you don't want everything broken down to a paste.

CAREFULLY remove the blade from the food processor. Divide the mixture into 4 equal patties. Arrange the patties on a plate and place them in the freezer for 20 minutes. (This will help them keep their shape during cooking.)

MEANWHILE, heat a grill to medium-high.

REMOVE the patties from the freezer and brush on both sides with the olive oil. Grill for 3 to 4 minutes per side, until grill marks develop and the falafel burgers are heated through. Alternatively, cook them in a skillet over medium-high heat for 3 to 4 minutes per side.

SERVE the falafel burgers on hamburger buns, with tomato, lettuce, and tzatziki, or store the patties in the fridge for up to 4 days and dress just before serving.

simple swaps

To makes these burgers vegan, simply swap out the egg for a flax egg (see page 19) and serve them without the tzatziki.

CAJUN RICE & BEANS

Cajun Rice & Beans are an absolute staple at our house, especially for Meatless Monday. This is one of those recipes that's so satisfying, it's always hard to believe that it's also completely vegan. Add the fact that it's loaded with fiber, protein, and veggies, and you've got a recipe for success. Oh, and did I mention that it's also made in a single pot? #winning

VEGETARIAN
VEGAN
WHEAT-FREE
DAIRY-FREE
PESCATARIAN

SERVINGS: **4**   PREP TIME: **10 MINUTES**   COOK TIME: **30 MINUTES**

---

1 tablespoon vegetable oil

1 small yellow onion, diced

3 celery stalks, diced

1 green bell pepper, diced

2 garlic cloves, minced

2 tablespoons Cajun Seasoning (page 231)

2 cups vegetable broth, homemade (page 204) or store-bought

1 (14.5-ounce) can diced tomatoes

1 (9-ounce) can red kidney beans, drained and rinsed

1 cup long-grain white rice

Salt and freshly ground black pepper

IN a large skillet with a tight-fitting lid, heat the vegetable oil over medium-high heat. Add the onion, celery, and bell pepper. Cook, stirring often, until they begin to soften, 4 to 5 minutes. Add the garlic and Cajun Seasoning and cook for 30 seconds more. Add the broth, tomatoes, kidney beans, and rice.

BRING the mixture to a boil, then reduce the heat to medium-low, cover, and simmer for 15 minutes. Turn off the heat and let sit for 5 minutes. Season with salt and pepper.

SERVE immediately or store in the refrigerator for up to 4 days.

mix it up

I have made this dish with shrimp, chicken, and cooked pork sausage. It never disappoints!

PAD THAI ZOODLES

DAIRY-FREE
PESCATARIAN

In the last few years, I've shared oodles of zoodle recipes on my YouTube channel, but none quite compare to these Pad Thai Zoodles. They're the perfect balance of sweet, tangy, and savory. If you've never made zoodles (zucchini noodles) before, I recommend skipping the overpriced spiralizer in favor of an inexpensive julienne peeler (see my Kitchen Essentials List on page 14 for more information).

SERVINGS: **14**　PREP TIME: **15 MINUTES**　COOK TIME: **15 MINUTES**

---

3 tablespoons fresh lime juice

3 tablespoons brown sugar

1 tablespoon soy sauce

2 teaspoons fish sauce

1 garlic clove, minced

½ teaspoon grated fresh ginger

¼ teaspoon red pepper flakes (optional)

2 tablespoons vegetable oil

8 ounces extra-firm tofu, cut into ¾-inch cubes

½ red bell pepper, julienned

1 medium carrot, julienned

3 large zucchini, julienned

1 cup bean sprouts

⅓ cup chopped peanuts

2 green onions, finely chopped

2 tablespoons fresh cilantro

1 lime, cut into wedges

IN a small bowl, whisk together the lime juice, brown sugar, soy sauce, fish sauce, garlic, ginger, and red pepper flakes (if using) until well combined.

IN a large wok or nonstick skillet, heat 1 tablespoon of the vegetable oil over medium-high heat. Add the tofu and cook, stirring often, until golden on all sides, 5 to 6 minutes. Remove the tofu from the skillet using a slotted spoon and transfer to a paper towel–lined plate.

IN the same skillet, heat the remaining 1 tablespoon oil, if necessary (there may be enough oil left in the pan). Add the bell pepper and carrot. Cook, stirring, until they begin to soften, about 3 minutes. Stir in the sauce and cooked tofu and cook for 2 minutes. Add the zucchini, bean sprouts, peanuts, and green onions. Toss well and cook until the zoodles have softened slightly and everything is heated through, about 3 minutes.

SERVE immediately, topped with the cilantro, with the lime wedges alongside.

simple swaps

The tofu in this recipe can be swapped out for 2 boneless, skinless chicken breasts, cut into ¾-inch cubes. Cook the chicken until golden on the outside and no longer pink inside, about 8 minutes.

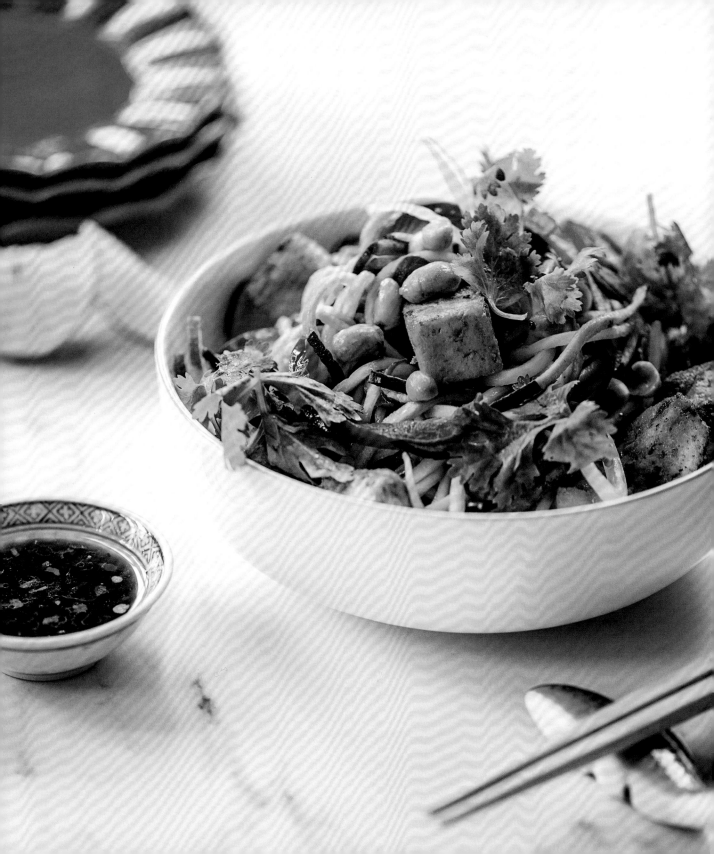

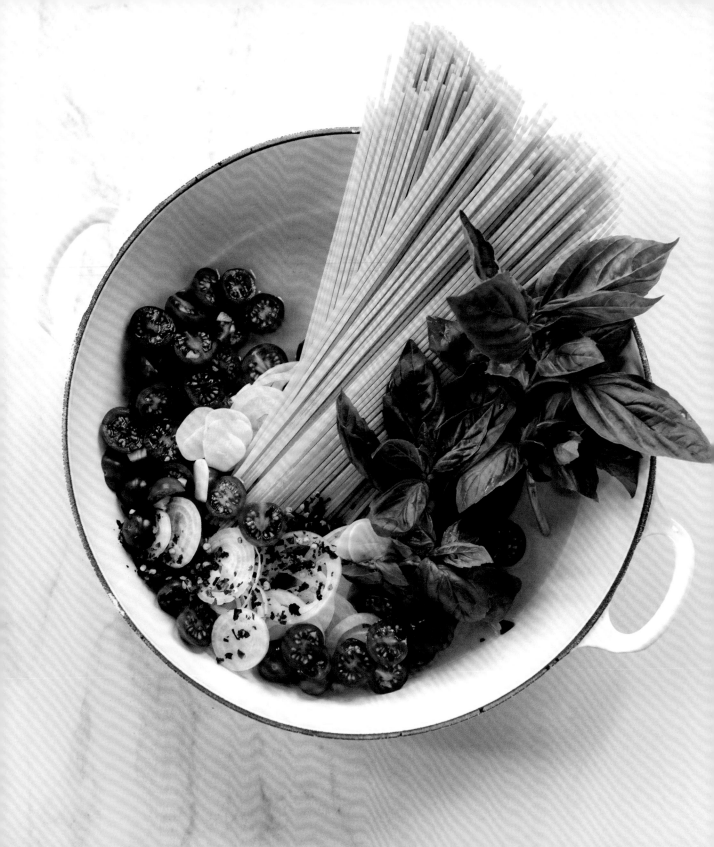

CLASSIC ONE-POT PASTA

It's fair to say that One-Pot Pasta has been nothing short of revolutionary, at least in my kitchen. The concept is simple: instead of cooking your pasta and your sauce in separate pots, you cook them together at the same time. The result is a richer, more flavorful dish with a much creamier texture than any traditional pasta could ever hope to achieve. The best part, beyond having just one pot to clean, is that once you've mastered the classic version, the flavor pasta-bilities are virtually endless.

SERVINGS: **6** PREP TIME: **5 MINUTES** COOK TIME: **15 MINUTES**

- **4 cups vegetable broth, homemade (page 204) or store-bought**
- **1 pound spaghetti**
- **2 cups halved cherry tomatoes**
- **1 small yellow onion, thinly sliced**
- **2 garlic cloves, minced**
- **5 fresh basil leaves**
- **½ teaspoon red pepper flakes (optional)**
- **Salt and freshly ground black pepper**
- **¼ cup freshly grated Parmesan cheese, for serving**

IN a large Dutch oven or soup pot with a tight-fitting lid, combine the broth, spaghetti, tomatoes, onion, garlic, basil, and red pepper flakes (if using). Bring the mixture to a boil over medium-high heat, then cover and reduce the heat to medium. Cook, stirring frequently, until all the liquid has been absorbed and the pasta is fully cooked, about 15 minutes. Season with salt and pepper.

SERVE immediately, topped with Parmesan, or let cool completely and store in the refrigerator for up to 3 days.

simple swaps

The vegetable broth in this recipe can easily be swapped out for chicken broth.

mix it up

As I mentioned earlier, there are countless variations on Classic One-Pot Pasta. Here are some of my very favorites . . .

ONE-POT MEDITERRANEAN PENNE

SERVINGS: **6**   PREP TIME: **10 MINUTES**   COOK TIME: **15 TO 20 MINUTES**

4 cups vegetable broth, homemade (page 204) or store-bought

1 pound penne

2 cups halved cherry tomatoes

2 garlic cloves, minced

1 tablespoon Greek Seasoning (page 230)

3 cups chopped baby spinach (4½ to 6 ounces)

½ cup chopped jarred artichoke hearts marinated in oil

¼ cup chopped jarred roasted red peppers

¼ cup chopped pitted Kalamata olives

Salt and freshly ground black pepper

¼ cup crumbled feta cheese, for serving

IN a large Dutch oven or soup pot with a tight-fitting lid, combine the broth, penne, tomatoes, garlic, and Greek Seasoning. Bring the mixture to a boil over medium-high heat, then cover and reduce the heat to medium. Cook, stirring frequently, until most of the liquid has been absorbed and the pasta is almost cooked through, about 15 minutes.

ADD the spinach, artichoke hearts, roasted red peppers, and olives and stir well. Cover and cook until the spinach has wilted and everything is heated through, about 2 minutes. Season with salt and pepper.

SERVE immediately, topped with the feta, or let cool completely and store in the refrigerator for up to 3 days.

simple swaps

The baby spinach in this recipe can easily be replaced with 2 cups finely chopped kale leaves.

ONE-POT CHILI CHEESE ROTINI

SERVINGS: **6**   PREP TIME: **10 MINUTES**   COOK TIME: **30 MINUTES**

1 tablespoon vegetable oil

1 small yellow onion, finely diced

1 pound extra-lean ground beef

1 (28-ounce) can diced tomatoes

3 cups chicken broth, homemade (page 206) or store-bought

1 (15-ounce) can red kidney beans, drained and rinsed

1 pound rotini

1 tablespoon chili powder

2 teaspoons ground cumin

2 teaspoons garlic powder

Salt and freshly ground black pepper

½ cup shredded sharp cheddar cheese

Sour cream, for serving

Minced fresh chives, for serving

IN a large Dutch oven or soup pot with a tight-fitting lid, heat the vegetable oil over medium-high heat. Add the onion and cook, stirring, until it begins to soften, 3 to 4 minutes. Add the ground beef and cook, breaking it up with a spoon as it browns, until cooked through, 6 to 8 minutes.

ADD the tomatoes, broth, kidney beans, rotini, chili powder, cumin, and garlic powder. Bring the mixture to a boil, then cover and reduce the heat to medium. Cook, stirring frequently, until all the liquid has been absorbed and the pasta is fully cooked, 12 to 14 minutes. Season with salt and pepper.

TURN off the heat and add the cheese. Stir until the cheese has completely melted.

SERVE immediately, with a dollop of sour cream and some chives, or let cool completely and store in the refrigerator for up to 3 days.

simple swaps

You can easily replace the ground beef in this recipe with ground turkey, ground chicken, or veggie crumbles.

ONE-POT CREAMY CHICKEN ALFREDO

SERVINGS: **6**　PREP TIME: **10 MINUTES**　COOK TIME: **25 MINUTES**

1 tablespoon vegetable oil

2 boneless, skinless chicken breasts, cut into ¾-inch cubes

Salt and freshly ground black pepper

4 cups chicken broth, homemade (page 206) or store-bought

1 pound fettuccine

1 cup 2% milk

2 garlic cloves, minced

½ cup freshly grated Parmesan cheese

2 tablespoons chopped fresh parsley

IN a large Dutch oven or soup pot with a tight-fitting lid, heat the vegetable oil over medium-high heat. Add the chicken and season with salt and pepper. Cook, stirring regularly, until the chicken is browned, 6 to 8 minutes.

ADD the broth, fettuccine, milk, and garlic. Bring the mixture to a boil, then cover and reduce the heat to medium. Cook, stirring frequently, until all the liquid has been absorbed and the pasta is fully cooked, about 15 minutes.

TURN off the heat and add the Parmesan and parsley. Stir until the Parmesan has melted. Season with salt and pepper.

SERVE immediately or let cool completely and store in the refrigerator for up to 3 days.

simple swaps

- If you want to make this dish even richer, go ahead and use heavy cream instead of the milk.
- If you'd prefer to keep this dish meatless, swap in some sliced mushrooms for the chicken, and vegetable broth for the chicken broth.

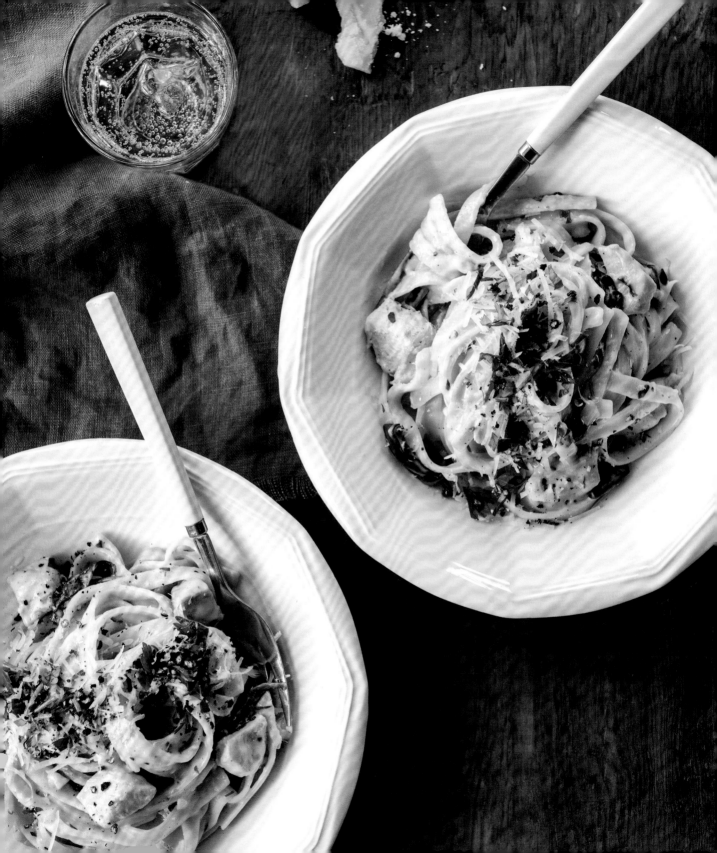

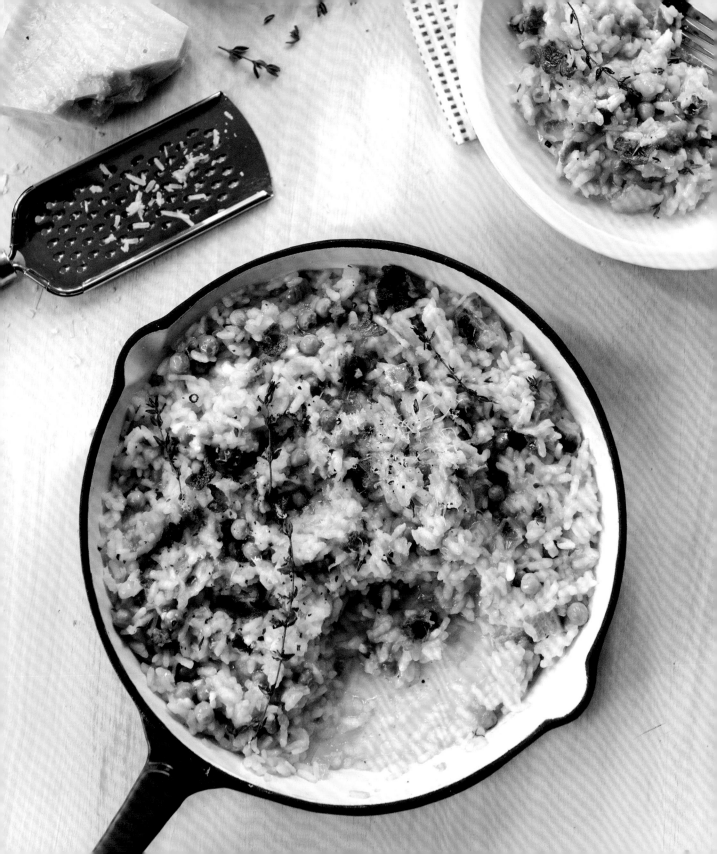

EASY-PEASY RISOTTO

WHEAT-FREE

If you've ever made a traditional risotto, you probably already know it's quite a labor of love. It typically requires standing over a skillet, stirring almost continuously, for nearly 30 minutes. And while I do simply adore risotto, I just don't have that kind of time (or patience) and I'm guessing you don't either. So I created my Easy-Peasy Risotto—all the creamy, dreamy deliciousness of traditional risotto with a lot less fuss.

SERVINGS: **4**   PREP TIME: **10 MINUTES**   COOK TIME: **35 MINUTES**

---

2 tablespoons butter

1 small yellow onion, diced

3 bacon slices, chopped

3 garlic cloves, minced

2 teaspoons fresh thyme leaves

2 cups Arborio rice

5 cups chicken broth, homemade (page 206) or store-bought

2 cups fresh or frozen shelled peas

½ cup freshly grated Parmesan cheese

Freshly ground black pepper

IN a large skillet with a lid, melt the butter over medium-high heat. Add the onion and cook, stirring, for 2 to 3 minutes. Add the bacon and cook, stirring, until the bacon is golden and crisp, about 6 minutes. Add the garlic, thyme, and rice and cook, stirring, until the rice becomes translucent and gives off a nutty aroma, 2 to 3 minutes.

ADD the broth and bring the mixture a boil, then cover the skillet and reduce the heat to medium-low. Cook, stirring often, until the liquid has been absorbed and the rice is tender, 18 to 20 minutes. Remove the lid and stir in the peas and Parmesan. Cook, stirring, until the Parmesan has been fully incorporated and the peas are heated through, 2 to 3 minutes. Season with pepper.

SERVE immediately or let cool completely and store in the refrigerator for up to 3 days. When it's time to reheat this dish, add a splash of chicken broth or water to help it rehydrate.

simple swaps

- The chicken broth in this dish can easily be swapped out for some vegetable or mushroom broth.
- Instead of bacon, try adding ½ cup chopped pancetta.

mix it up

MUSHROOM-SPINACH RISOTTO

Replace the bacon in this dish with 2 cups chopped mushrooms. Add them to the skillet with the onions and cook until they are soft and golden, about 6 minutes. Replace the peas with 2 cups chopped baby spinach (3 to 4 ounces).

MEDITERRANEAN CHICKEN LEGS

In the kitchen, as in life, simple is so often best, and that's definitely the case with this delicious dish. It's not fussy or difficult to prepare, but the flavors just speak for themselves. I should also mention that this is the recipe my husband requests most often in my house. He loves a classic!

SERVINGS: **4**   PREP TIME: **1 HOUR 10 MINUTES**   COOK TIME: **45 MINUTES**

¼ cup extra-virgin olive oil

2 garlic cloves, minced

Grated zest and juice of 1 lemon

2 tablespoons Greek Seasoning (page 230)

2 tablespoons chopped fresh parsley

Salt and freshly ground black pepper

4 whole chicken legs

IN a small bowl, combine the olive oil, garlic, lemon zest, lemon juice, Greek Seasoning, parsley, and salt and pepper. Whisk well. Place the chicken legs in a zipper bag and pour over the marinade. Seal the bag and shake until the chicken legs are evenly coated. Marinate in the refrigerator for at least 1 hour but ideally overnight.

WHEN it's time to cook the chicken, preheat the oven to 375°F.

TRANSFER the chicken to an oven-safe baking dish. Bake until it's golden on top and a meat thermometer inserted into the thickest part registers 165°F, about 40 minutes. Switch the oven to the broil setting and broil until the chicken skin becomes crisp and golden, about 4 minutes.

SERVE immediately or let cool completely and store in the refrigerator for up to 3 days.

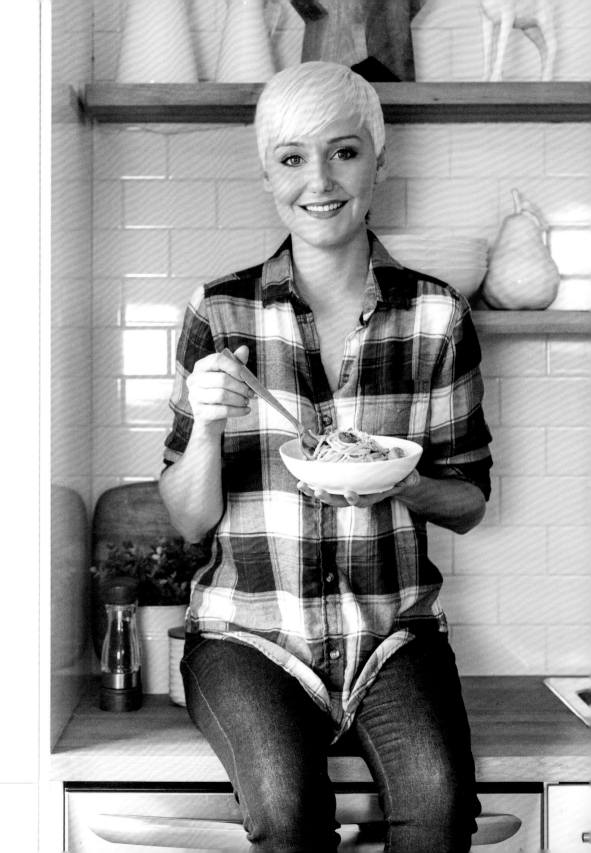

BAKED GARLIC SHRIMP

WHEAT-FREE
PESCATARIAN

I know this is a bold statement, but Baked Garlic Shrimp is my absolute favorite weeknight meal. In fact, I can't think of a dinner dish that is easier to make while also being so delicious. The most amazing part is that it uses the simplest ingredients, but the results taste totally gourmet. There will be plenty of flavorful liquid left over in the bottom of the baking dish, so pour it over cooked rice, pasta, or even on a salad. Or just sop it up with crusty French bread.

SERVINGS: **4**   PREP TIME: **5 MINUTES**   COOK TIME: **8 TO 10 MINUTES**

---

2 pounds large shrimp, peeled and deveined

¼ cup white wine

3 garlic cloves, minced

Grated zest and juice of ½ lemon

½ teaspoon red pepper flakes (optional)

Salt and freshly ground black pepper

2 tablespoons butter, cubed

Chopped fresh parsley, for garnish

PREHEAT the oven to 425°F.

ARRANGE the shrimp in an even layer in an oven-safe baking dish. Top with the wine, garlic, lemon zest, lemon juice, red pepper flakes (if using), and salt and pepper. Arrange the butter cubes evenly on top of the shrimp. Bake until the shrimp turn pink and opaque, 8 to 10 minutes.

SERVE immediately, garnished with parsley, or store in the refrigerator for up to 3 days.

mix it up

You can switch up the flavor profile of this dish by simply changing the seasonings—try adding 1 tablespoon of my Greek, Italian, or Cajun Seasonings (pages 230 and 231) to this recipe before baking.

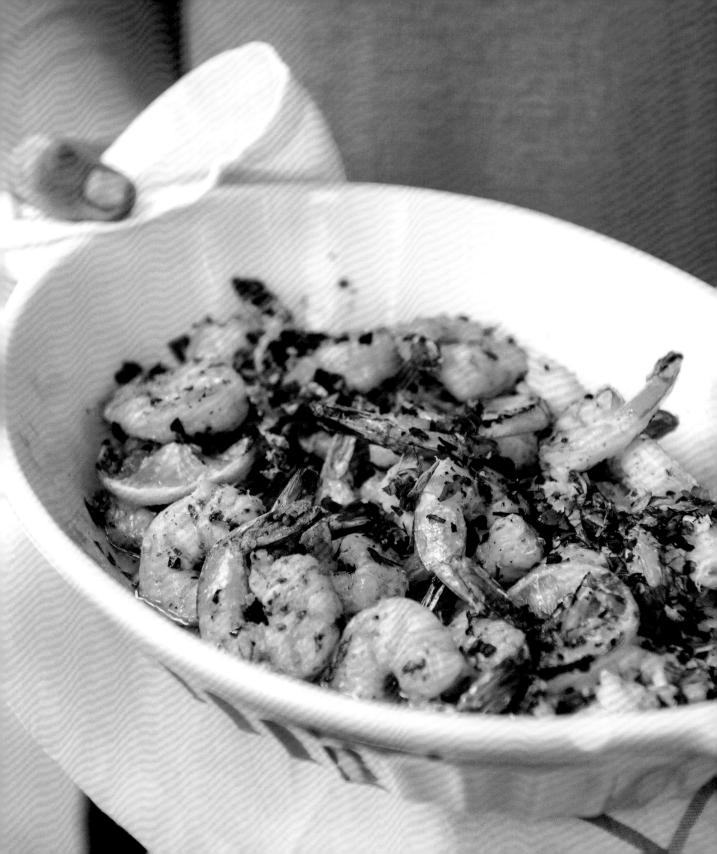

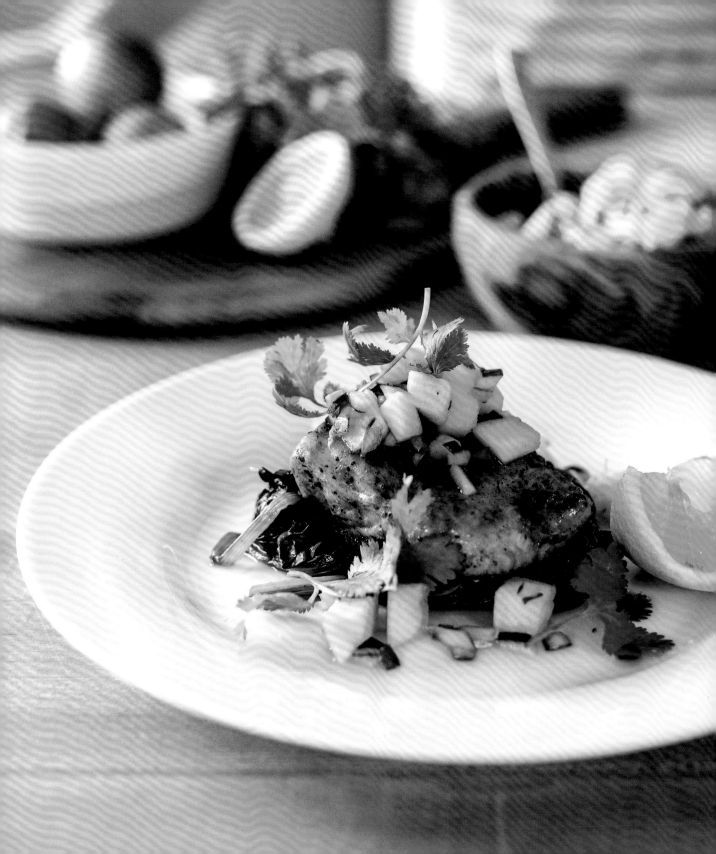

MAHI-MAHI WITH FRESH PINEAPPLE SALSA

WHEAT-FREE
DAIRY-FREE
PESCATARIAN

This light, fruity dinner idea is really refreshing on a warm summer evening. It comes together in a flash, which hopefully means less time in the kitchen and more time on the patio. I like to pair it with a nice glass of white wine, because why not?

SERVINGS: **4**   PREP TIME: **3 MINUTES**   COOK TIME: **6 MINUTES**

---

4 (4-ounce) mahi-mahi fillets

2 tablespoons Cajun Seasoning (page 231)

Salt and freshly ground black pepper

1 tablespoon vegetable oil

2 cups Pineapple Salsa (page 217)

Lemon or lime wedges, for serving

PAT the fish fillets dry with a paper towel. Season each fillet on both sides with the Cajun Seasoning and salt and pepper. Gently rub the seasoning in to coat the fish.

IN a large skillet, heat the vegetable oil over medium-high heat. Add the fish in a single layer (do not overcrowd the pan—cook in batches, if necessary) and cook until a crust starts to form on the first side, about 3 minutes. Flip the fillets and cook until they're firm and flake easily with a fork, about 3 minutes more.

SERVE immediately, topped with pineapple salsa and with lemon or lime wedges alongside, or store in the refrigerator for up to 3 days.

simple swaps

While mahi-mahi is absolutely delicious, other fish certainly work in this recipe. You could try some tilapia or snapper, or even swap in some salmon. Each will have a slightly different taste and texture, but variety is the spice of life.

SPICY SAUSAGE, KALE & POTATO SOUP

This hearty soup totally eats like a meal thanks to lots of spicy Italian sausage and filling russet potatoes. And it's so flavorful that you might not even notice the abundance of kale hidden in it. Seriously though, if you've got picky eaters in your household who are reluctant to eat their greens, this delicious soup might just be the answer.

SERVINGS: **6**   PREP TIME: **5 MINUTES**   COOK TIME: **40 MINUTES**

---

1 tablespoon extra-virgin olive oil

1 small yellow onion, finely diced

2 garlic cloves, minced

1 pound hot Italian sausage, casings removed

8 cups chicken broth, homemade (page 206) or store-bought

5 cups finely chopped kale leaves

2 large russet potatoes, peeled and diced

1 (14.5-ounce) can diced tomatoes

Salt and freshly ground black pepper

IN a large Dutch oven or soup pot, heat the olive oil over medium-high heat. Add the onion and cook, stirring, until soft and translucent, about 3 minutes. Stir in the garlic and cook until fragrant, about 30 seconds. Add the sausage and cook, breaking it up with the spoon as it cooks, until it's no longer pink, 6 to 8 minutes. Add the broth, kale, potatoes, and tomatoes and stir to combine.

BRING the soup to a boil, then reduce the heat to medium, cover, and simmer until the potatoes are tender, 20 to 25 minutes. Season the soup with salt and pepper.

SERVE hot, or let cool and store in the refrigerator for up to 3 days or in the freezer for up to 3 months.

simple swaps

To make this soup vegan, swap out the hot Italian sausage for 1 pound sliced vegan sausage and the chicken broth for vegetable broth. Add ½ teaspoon red pepper flakes with the salt and pepper for additional heat.

VEGETARIAN WHITE BEAN CASSOULET

This lightened-up vegetarian version of a classic French cassoulet takes a fraction of the time but still results in incredible flavor that easily rivals the original dish. It's just a bit more time-consuming than most of the dinners in this chapter, but still really easy to make. I recommend saving this one for a special Sunday supper. It's one of those recipes you have to taste to believe.

SERVINGS: **4** PREP TIME: **10 MINUTES** COOK TIME: **45 TO 50 MINUTES**

2 tablespoons butter

3 leeks, thinly sliced crosswise and well rinsed

2 celery stalks, finely diced

2 medium carrots, finely diced

1 parsnip, peeled and finely diced

3 garlic cloves, minced

4 cups vegetable broth, homemade (page 204) or store-bought

2 (15-ounce) cans navy beans, drained and rinsed

2 fresh thyme sprigs

1 fresh rosemary sprig

1 bay leaf

Salt and freshly ground black pepper

½ cup bread crumbs

¼ cup chopped fresh parsley

Grated zest of 1 lemon

2 tablespoons extra-virgin olive oil

IN a large Dutch oven or deep oven-safe skillet, melt the butter over medium-high heat. Add the leeks, celery, carrots, and parsnip and cook, stirring often, until they begin to soften, about 6 minutes. Add the garlic and cook, stirring, for about 30 seconds. Add the broth, navy beans, thyme, rosemary, and bay leaf.

BRING the mixture to a boil, then reduce the heat to medium and simmer until most of the liquid has been evaporated and the mixture has a stew-like consistency, about 20 minutes. Remove and discard the thyme and rosemary sprigs and the bay leaf. Season liberally with salt and pepper.

MEANWHILE, preheat the oven to 350°F.

IN a small bowl, combine the bread crumbs, parsley, lemon zest, and olive oil. Crumble the mixture over the top of the cassoulet and bake until the top is golden brown, 15 to 20 minutes, broiling for the final 2 minutes.

THIS dish is best enjoyed hot, straight out of the oven. If you're making it in advance, I recommend preparing the stew portion only, without the bread crumb topping, and refrigerating it for up to 4 days. Reheat the stew over medium heat in a Dutch oven or oven-safe skillet, then add the bread crumb topping and bake as directed.

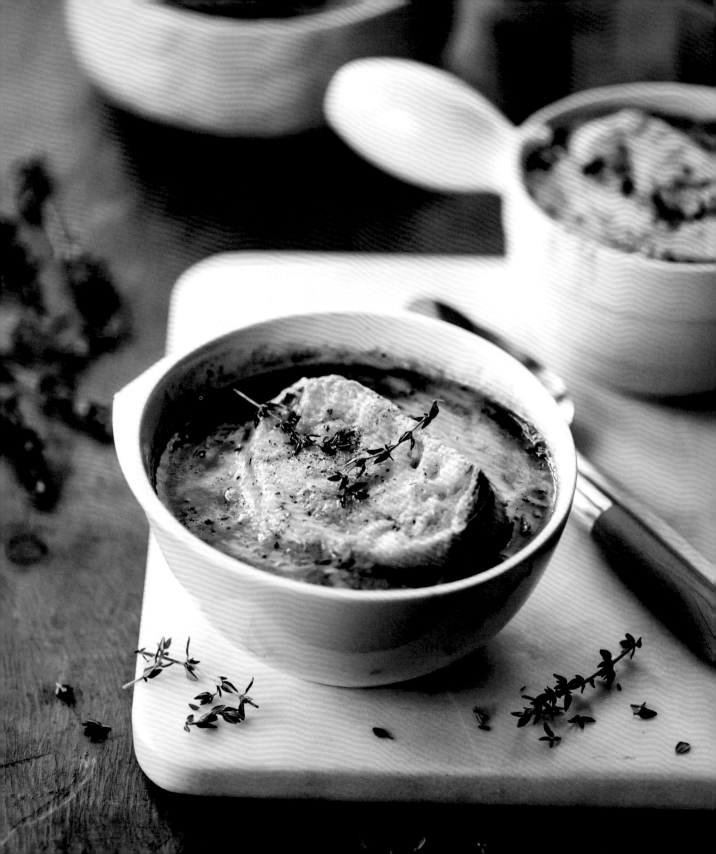

CLASSIC FRENCH ONION SOUP

As far as I'm concerned, French Onion Soup is the ultimate weekend comfort food, and even though it's deeply flavorful, it's surprisingly easy to make. It starts with a hearty, slow-simmered onion-and-beef broth that's then topped with crusty toasted baguette, smothered in cheese, and baked until it has reached its ooey-gooey-ist. This classic French recipe is definitely on the richer side, but worth each and every calorie.

SERVINGS: **4**   PREP TIME: **15 MINUTES**   COOK TIME: **1 HOUR 15 MINUTES**

---

2 tablespoons butter

6 large onions, thinly sliced

Salt and freshly ground black pepper

2 tablespoons all-purpose flour

⅔ cup red wine

8 cups beef broth

3 fresh thyme sprigs, plus more for garnish

1 French baguette, cut into ½-inch-thick slices

1 cup shredded Gruyère cheese

IN a large Dutch oven or soup pot, melt the butter over medium heat. Add the onions and stir until they are well coated with the butter. Cover the Dutch oven and cook until the onions begin to soften, about 10 minutes. Remove the lid and season the onions with salt and pepper. Cook, stirring occasionally, until the onions are a deep, golden brown, about 20 minutes.

STIR in the flour and cook for another minute. Add the wine and cook, stirring, for 2 to 3 minutes more. Add the broth and thyme and bring the mixture to a boil, then reduce the heat to medium-low, cover, and simmer for 30 minutes.

WHILE the soup is simmering, preheat the oven to 375°F.

ARRANGE the baguette slices on a baking sheet and bake until crisp, about 10 minutes. Remove the baguette slices from the oven and set aside.

ONCE the soup is finished simmering, use a slotted spoon to carefully remove and discard the thyme sprigs.

SET four individual oven-safe bowls on a rimmed baking sheet. Ladle the soup into the bowls and top each with 2 toasted baguette slices and 2 tablespoons of the Gruyère. Bake until the cheese is melted, golden, and bubbling, about 6 minutes.

SERVE immediately, hot from the oven. The soup, without the baguette and cheese topping, can be stored in the refrigerator for up to 4 days. Reheat the soup, then top with the baguette slices and cheese, and bake as directed just before serving. Garnish with thyme sprigs.

simple swaps

- The red wine in this recipe can easily be swapped out for more beef broth, if desired.
- When I'm entertaining vegetarian guests, I use my homemade Vegetable Broth (page 204) in place of beef broth. I also add 2 tablespoons soy sauce.

EASY ROAST CHICKEN

WHEAT-FREE

DAIRY-FREE

Whether I'm hosting family dinner or just doing my weekly meal prep, roasting a chicken is a Sunday must at my house. There are few dishes more comforting than a whole roasted chicken, and even if you're only cooking for one or two, having some leftover chicken in the fridge is a great way to make weeknight cooking a lot less daunting. It can be added to soups, stews, chilies, salads, sandwiches—the list goes on and on. Here is my foolproof roast chicken recipe that will make your life easier each and every week . . .

SERVINGS: **4**   PREP TIME: **5 MINUTES**   COOK TIME: **1 HOUR 35 MINUTES**

1 (4-pound) chicken

1 small lemon, quartered

4 garlic cloves, smashed

6 fresh thyme sprigs

2 fresh rosemary sprigs

3 tablespoons extra-virgin olive oil

1 teaspoon garlic powder

Salt and freshly ground black pepper

PREHEAT the oven to 450°F.

PLACE the chicken, breast-side up, in a roasting pan. Pat it dry with a paper towel to remove excess moisture. Stuff the cavity with the lemon, garlic, thyme, and rosemary. Drizzle the chicken with the olive oil and season it liberally all over with the garlic powder and salt and pepper.

PLACE the chicken in the oven and reduce the oven temperature to 400°F. Bake until the chicken is golden brown and a meat thermometer inserted into the inner thigh (without touching bone) registers 165°F, about 1 hour 30 minutes. Switch the oven to the broil setting and broil until the chicken skin is crisp and golden, about 4 minutes. Keep a close eye on it to ensure it doesn't burn.

REMOVE the chicken from the oven, tent it with aluminum foil, and let rest for 10 minutes before carving.

SERVE immediately or store in the refrigerator for up to 3 days.

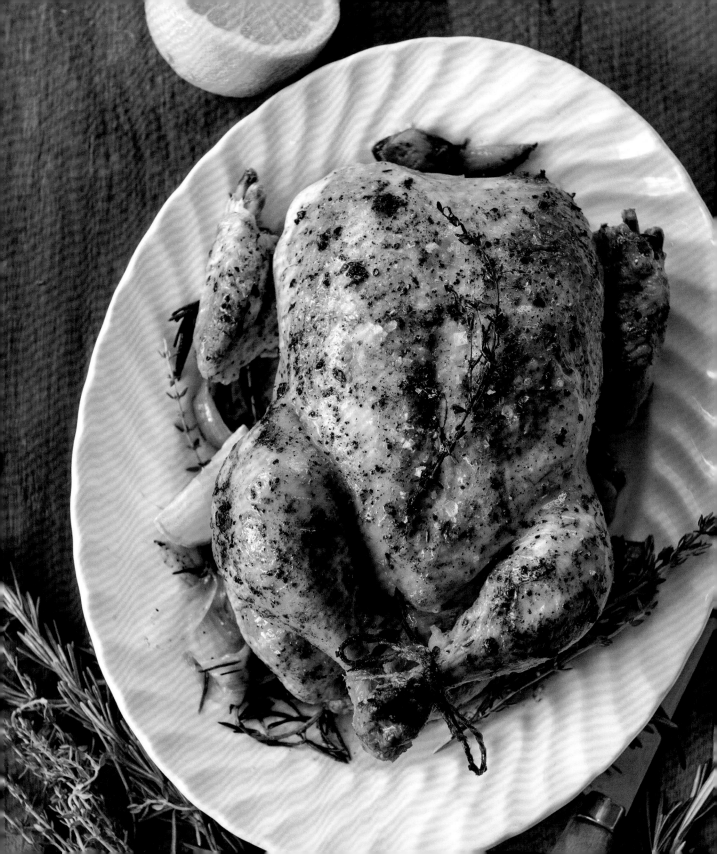

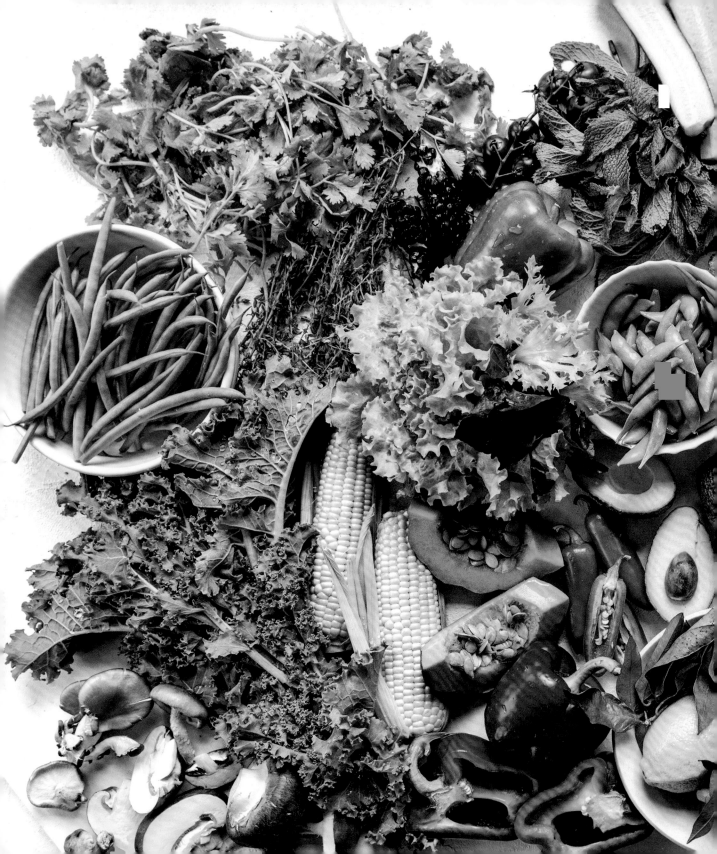

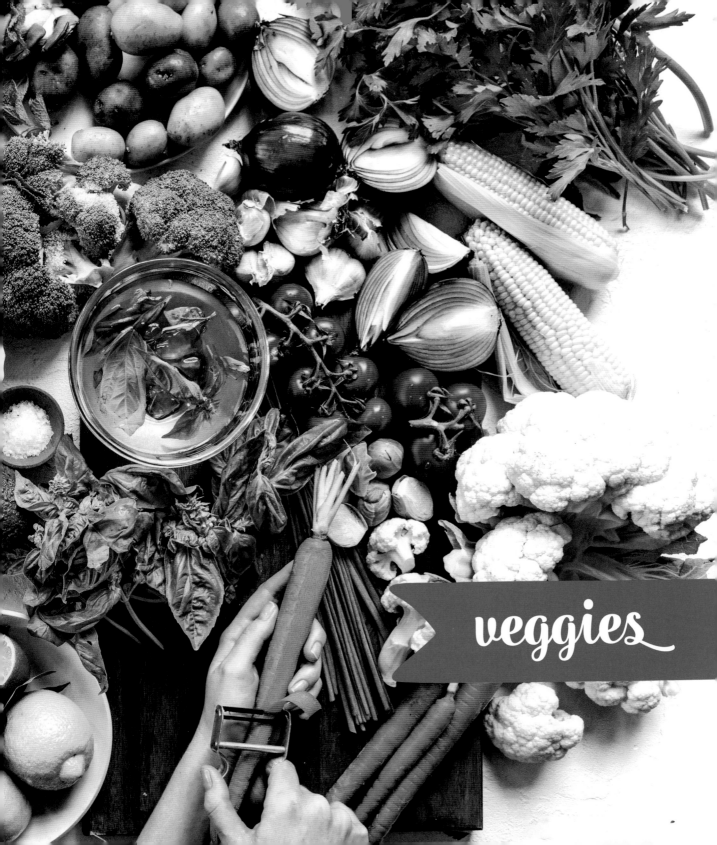

veggies

FRESH GREEN BEAN SALAD

VEGETARIAN
WHEAT-FREE
PESCATARIAN

Green beans are actually my favorite veggie. I love their vibrant color, crisp bite, and naturally sweet taste. This simple salad is effortless to make but so flavorful you won't be able to get enough. I recommend serving it with Baked Garlic Shrimp (page 168) and dining alfresco.

SERVINGS: **4**   PREP TIME: **10 MINUTES**   COOK TIME: **4 MINUTES**

3 tablespoons extra-virgin olive oil

2 tablespoons red wine vinegar

1 tablespoon minced shallot

1 teaspoon chopped fresh tarragon

Salt and freshly ground black pepper

2 pounds green beans, trimmed

1 cup halved cherry tomatoes

¼ cup crumbled feta cheese

IN a small bowl, whisk together the olive oil, vinegar, shallot, tarragon, and salt and pepper.

BRING a large pot of water to a boil. Add the green beans and cook until they are bright green and tender, 3 to 4 minutes. Transfer the green beans to a large bowl of ice water to stop the cooking. Let cool, then drain them and blot dry with paper towels.

ARRANGE the green beans and cherry tomatoes in a serving dish. Pour the vinaigrette over the beans and tomatoes and toss. Top with the feta.

SERVE immediately or store in the refrigerator for up to 4 days.

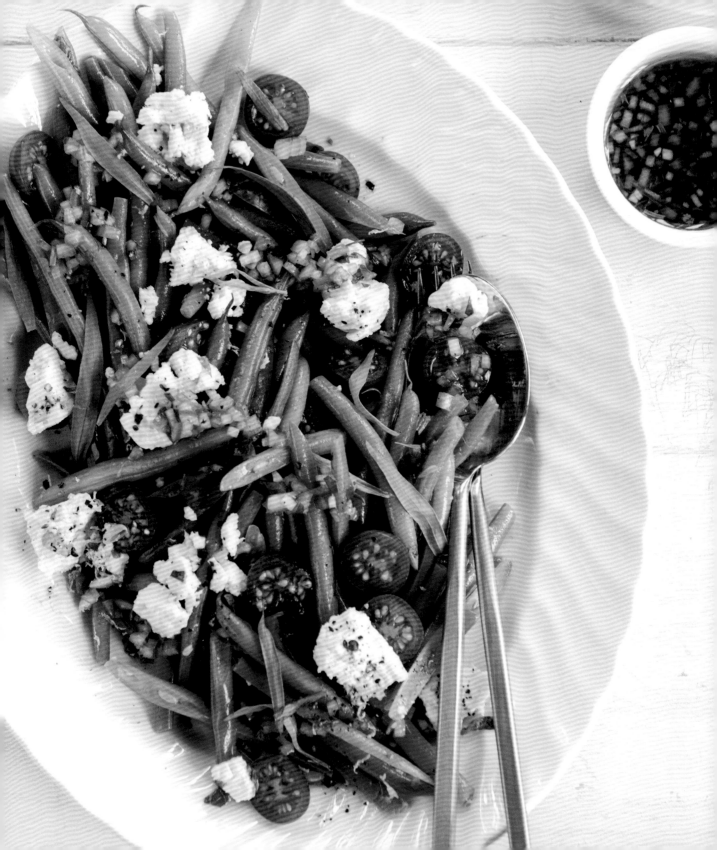

CHILI-GARLIC BROCCOLI

VEGETARIAN
WHEAT-FREE
PESCATARIAN

This recipe is a gloriously garlicky way to make your broccoli something special. I love serving it as a side dish with my incredibly easy Better-Than-Takeout Orange Chicken (page 132).

SERVINGS: **4**   PREP TIME: **5 MINUTES**   COOK TIME: **7 MINUTES**

1 tablespoon butter

3 garlic cloves, thinly sliced

1 red chile, thinly sliced

6 cups small broccoli florets

¼ cup water

Salt and freshly ground black pepper

IN a large skillet with a tight-fitting lid, melt the butter over medium-high heat. Add the garlic and chile and cook, stirring, until the garlic is lightly golden, 1 to 2 minutes. Add the broccoli and toss. Add the water, cover, and cook until the broccoli is bright green and tender but still a little crisp, about 5 minutes. Season with salt and pepper.

SERVE immediately or store in the refrigerator for up to 4 days.

simple swaps

If you're not a fan of the heat, skip the chile and add the grated zest and juice of ½ lemon instead.

CREAMED SPINACH

This Popeye-approved side dish is rich, creamy, and surprisingly satisfying, considering it's loaded with the good stuff. Dish it up with the Mediterranean Chicken Legs on page 166, and you've got yourself some dinner.

SERVINGS: **4**   PREP TIME: **5 MINUTES**   COOK TIME: **10 MINUTES**

1 pound frozen chopped spinach, defrosted

1 tablespoon butter

1 small yellow onion, finely diced

2 garlic cloves, minced

1 tablespoon all-purpose flour

½ cup 2% milk

2 tablespoons cream cheese

⅛ teaspoon grated nutmeg

2 tablespoons freshly grated Parmesan cheese

½ teaspoon red pepper flakes (optional)

Salt and freshly ground black pepper

REMOVE the excess liquid from the thawed spinach by squeezing it in small handfuls over a colander or by placing the spinach in a clean kitchen towel, gathering the sides, and twisting to squeeze out the moisture. Set aside.

IN a large cast-iron skillet, melt the butter over medium-high heat. Add the onion and cook, stirring, until it begins to soften, about 4 minutes. Stir in the garlic and cook until it becomes fragrant, about 30 seconds. Add the flour and cook, stirring continuously, for another minute.

REDUCE the heat to medium-low and slowly stir in the milk. Cook until the milk is heated through, then stir in the cream cheese and cook until the mixture has thickened. Add the spinach, nutmeg, and Parmesan and mix well. Cook until the spinach is heated through. Season the spinach with the red pepper flakes (if using) and salt and pepper.

SERVE immediately or store in the refrigerator for up to 3 days.

mix it up

Creamed Spinach makes a delicious addition to breakfast. Divide it among four individual oven-safe dishes and crack an egg on top of each. Bake for 8 to 10 minutes, or until the eggs are cooked to your liking.

PARMESAN ROASTED CAULIFLOWER

Cauliflower is such a versatile veggie, which is why it's so beloved in my household. There are dozens of clever ways to prepare it, but for me, nothing is more effortless than tossing it with a little extra-virgin olive oil, salt, and pepper and roasting it until it's golden. A sprinkle of freshly grated Parmesan cheese takes it from good to can't-get-enough.

SERVINGS: **4**   PREP TIME: **5 MINUTES**   COOK TIME: **35 MINUTES**

---

1 large head cauliflower, cut into florets

2 tablespoons extra-virgin olive oil

Salt and freshly ground black pepper

½ cup freshly grated Parmesan cheese

2 tablespoons freshly chopped parsley

PREHEAT the oven to 375°F.

ARRANGE the cauliflower on a large baking sheet and drizzle with the olive oil. Season with salt and pepper and toss well. Bake for 25 to 30 minutes, tossing once, until the cauliflower has softened and is slightly golden. Sprinkle with the Parmesan and bake for 3 to 5 minutes more, until the Parmesan is melted and lightly golden.

SERVE immediately, garnished with the fresh parsley.

mix it up

In addition to the salt and pepper, try tossing the cauliflower with 1 teaspoon Italian Seasoning (page 230) and ½ teaspoon red pepper flakes before roasting. It makes the perfect side for my Healthy Chicken Piccata (page 131).

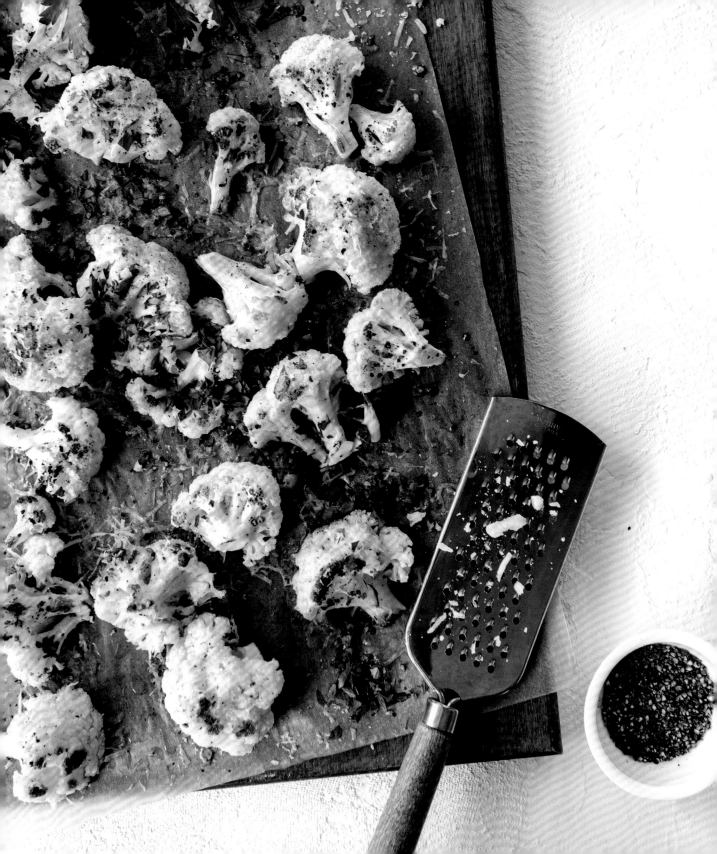

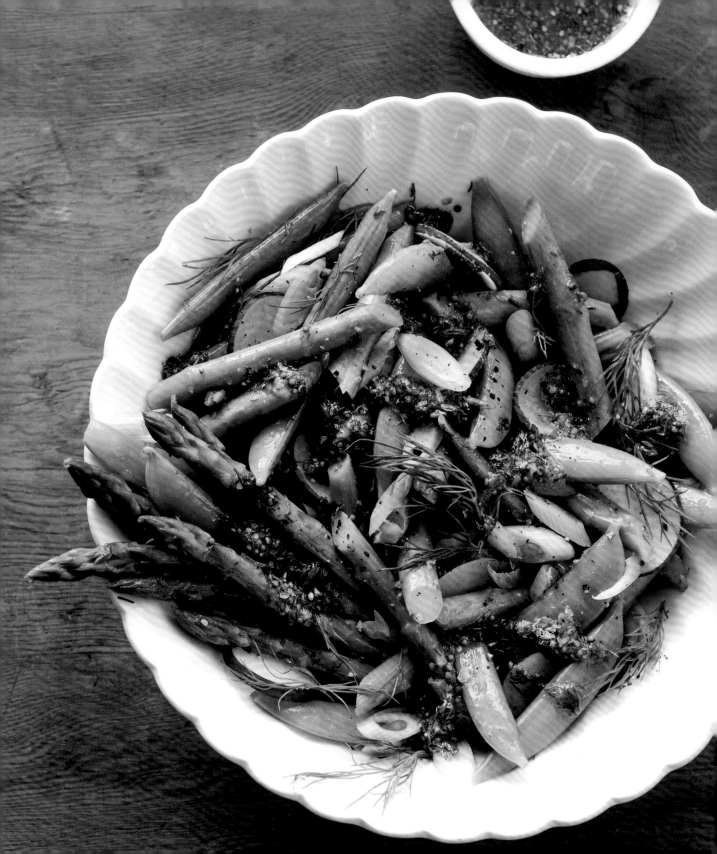

CRUNCHY SPRING VEGETABLES

VEGETARIAN

VEGAN

WHEAT-FREE

DAIRY-FREE

PESCATARIAN

This fresh, flavorful side is a great way to celebrate the arrival of spring. With its crisp texture and tangy vinaigrette, these Crunchy Spring Vegetables are guaranteed to be love at first bite. This dish pairs perfectly with the Classic Lemon & Dill Salmon on page 136.

SERVINGS: **4**   PREP TIME: **10 MINUTES**   COOK TIME: **5 MINUTES**

2 tablespoons extra-virgin olive oil

2 tablespoons white wine vinegar

1 tablespoon grainy Dijon mustard

Salt and freshly ground black pepper

1 pound asparagus, cut into 2-inch pieces

2 cups sugar snap peas, strings removed

1 cup thinly sliced radishes

¼ cup thinly sliced green onions

2 tablespoons chopped fresh dill

IN a small bowl, whisk together the olive oil, vinegar, mustard, and salt and pepper. Set it aside.

FILL a large pot fitted with a steamer basket with 1 inch of water. Bring the water to a simmer over medium-high heat. Put the asparagus in the steamer basket, cover the pot, and steam for 1 to 2 minutes, or until the asparagus is bright green. Add the snap peas and steam for 1 to 2 minutes more, until the snap peas are bright green and still crunchy. Transfer the steamed vegetables to a bowl of ice water to stop the cooking and let cool completely. Drain the vegetables and transfer to a large bowl. Add the radishes, green onions, and dill. Pour over the vinaigrette and toss to coat the vegetables. Season with salt and pepper.

SERVE immediately or store in the refrigerator for up to 3 days.

CREAMY KALE SLAW

VEGETARIAN
WHEAT-FREE
PESCATARIAN

This cool, creamy, crunchy slaw is really refreshing and full of good-for-you ingredients like carrots, red cabbage, and kale. If you're not usually a kale fan, don't fret. Finely chopping the kale and softening it in this sweet-and-tart dressing makes it a lot more palatable. Pair it with the Falafel Burgers on page 154, and you've got a great menu for outdoor entertaining.

SERVINGS: **4**   PREP TIME: **10 MINUTES**

½ cup plain Greek yogurt

Grated zest and juice of 1 lemon

1 tablespoon grainy Dijon mustard

1 tablespoon honey

1 teaspoon caraway seeds

Salt and freshly ground black pepper

4 cups finely chopped kale leaves

2 cups finely chopped red cabbage

2 medium carrots, shredded

½ small red onion, finely sliced

IN a small bowl, whisk together the yogurt, lemon zest, lemon juice, mustard, honey, and caraway. Season with salt and pepper.

IN a large bowl, combine the kale, cabbage, carrots, and onion and toss well. Pour the dressing over the kale mixture and toss again until everything is evenly dressed.

SERVE immediately or store in the refrigerator for up to 4 days.

simple swaps

If you're really not a fan of kale, feel free to swap in some crunchy green cabbage instead for a more traditional coleslaw.

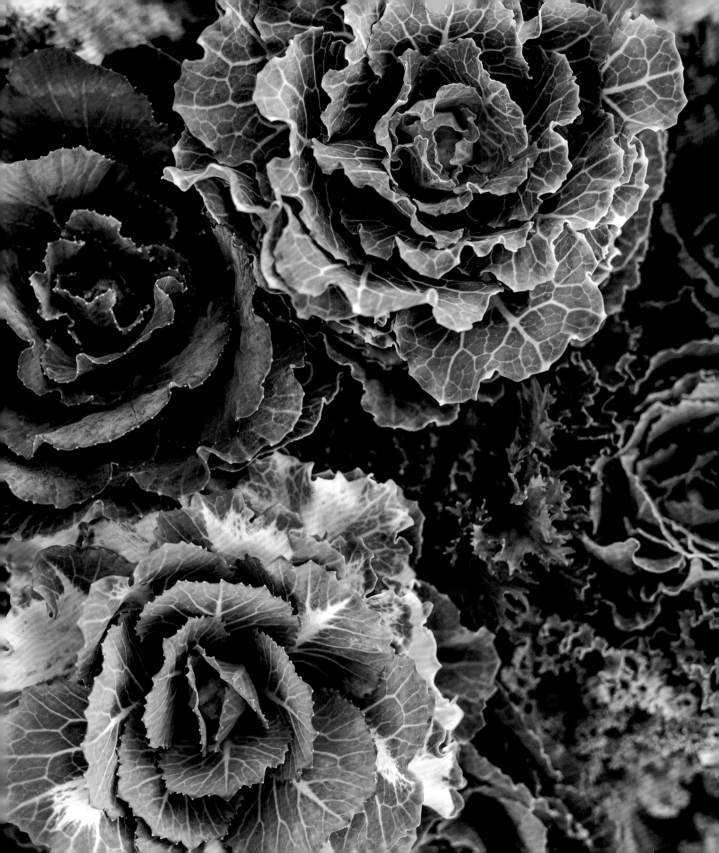

SWEET CORN SALAD

VEGETARIAN
WHEAT-FREE
PESCATARIAN

For me, this Sweet Corn Salad is the epitome of a summer side dish. The sweetness of seasonal corn is beautifully complemented by a tangy vinaigrette and some savory crumbled feta cheese. Plus, this dish gets plenty of crunch and flavor from other summer faves like cucumber, tomato, and fresh basil.

SERVINGS: **4**   PREP TIME: **10 MINUTES**   COOK TIME: **5 MINUTES**

---

5 ears corn, shucked

1 cup halved cherry tomatoes

1 cup finely diced cucumber

¼ cup chopped green onions

2 tablespoons extra-virgin olive oil

2 tablespoons white wine vinegar

2 tablespoons chopped fresh basil leaves

Salt and freshly ground black pepper

¼ cup crumbled feta cheese

BRING a large pot of water to a boil. Add the corn and cook until the kernels have turned bright yellow, about 5 minutes. Drain and transfer the corn to a large bowl of ice water to stop the cooking. Let cool completely, then carefully cut the kernels from each cob with a serrated knife.

TRANSFER the corn to a large bowl and add the tomatoes, cucumber, green onions, olive oil, vinegar, and basil. Toss to combine. Season with salt and pepper and toss again. Top the salad with the feta.

SERVE immediately or store in the refrigerator for up to 4 days.

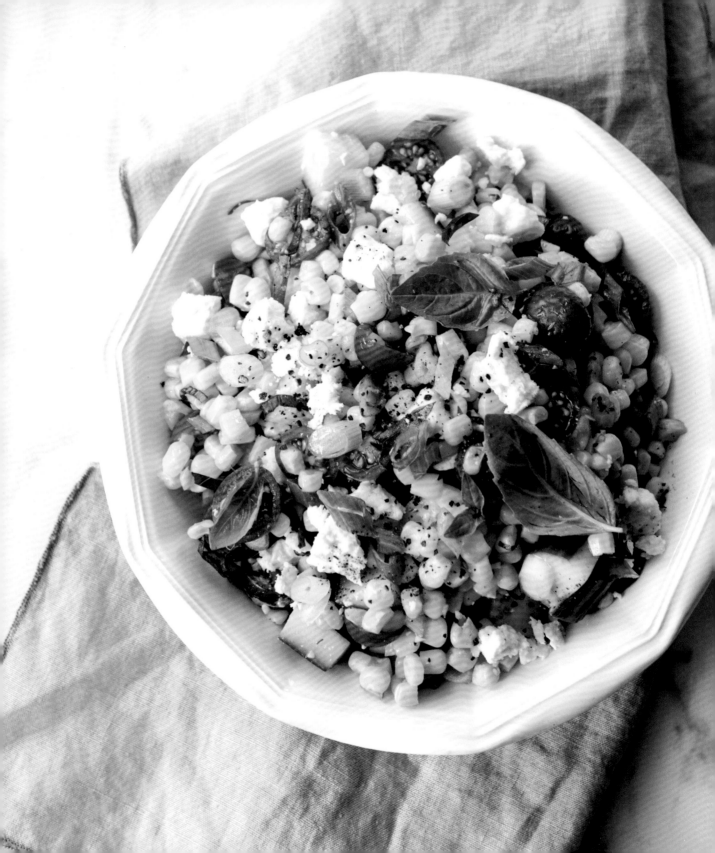

GARLIC & HERB ROASTED POTATOES

VEGETARIAN
VEGAN
WHEAT-FREE
DAIRY-FREE
PESCATARIAN

Simple roasted potatoes are a comforting classic, but add some garlic and fresh herbs, and you've got a side dish that will have everyone asking for seconds. This yumminess pairs beautifully with the Balsamic-Glazed Chicken on page 135.

SERVINGS: **6**   PREP TIME: **5 MINUTES**   COOK TIME: **40 MINUTES**

5 large white or red potatoes, diced

2 tablespoons extra-virgin olive oil

1 tablespoon finely chopped fresh rosemary leaves

1 teaspoon garlic powder

Salt and freshly ground black pepper

2 tablespoons finely chopped fresh parsley

PREHEAT the oven to 400°F. Line a baking sheet with parchment paper.

IN a large bowl, toss the potatoes with the olive oil, rosemary, garlic powder, and salt and pepper. Transfer the potatoes to the prepared baking sheet and arrange them in an even layer. Bake, tossing twice during cooking, until the potatoes are tender and golden, 35 to 40 minutes.

SERVE immediately, topped with the fresh parsley, or let cool completely and store in the refrigerator for up to 3 days. For best results, reheat the potatoes on a baking sheet in the oven before serving.

simple swaps

Replace the chopped rosemary and garlic powder in this recipe with 1 tablespoon Italian Seasoning (page 230), Greek Seasoning (page 230), or Cajun Seasoning (page 231).

MAPLE ROASTED SQUASH

This slightly sweet side dish is inspired by the lovely flavors of fall. It's the perfect accompaniment to my Easy Roast Chicken (page 176). Sunday dinner is served.

SERVINGS: **4**   PREP TIME: **5 MINUTES**   COOK TIME: **30 MINUTES**

1 large acorn squash, halved lengthwise and seeded (do not peel)

1 tablespoon extra-virgin olive oil

Salt and freshly ground black pepper

2 tablespoons maple syrup

1 tablespoon chopped fresh sage

PREHEAT the oven to 400°F.

CUT each squash in half crosswise into ¼-inch-thick slices. Transfer the squash to a large bowl and toss with the olive oil and salt and pepper. Arrange the squash on a large baking sheet and bake for 20 to 25 minutes, until tender. Remove from the oven (keep the oven on) and brush each slice with the maple syrup. Top with the sage. Return to the oven and bake for 5 minutes more.

SERVE immediately or store in the refrigerator for up to 3 days.

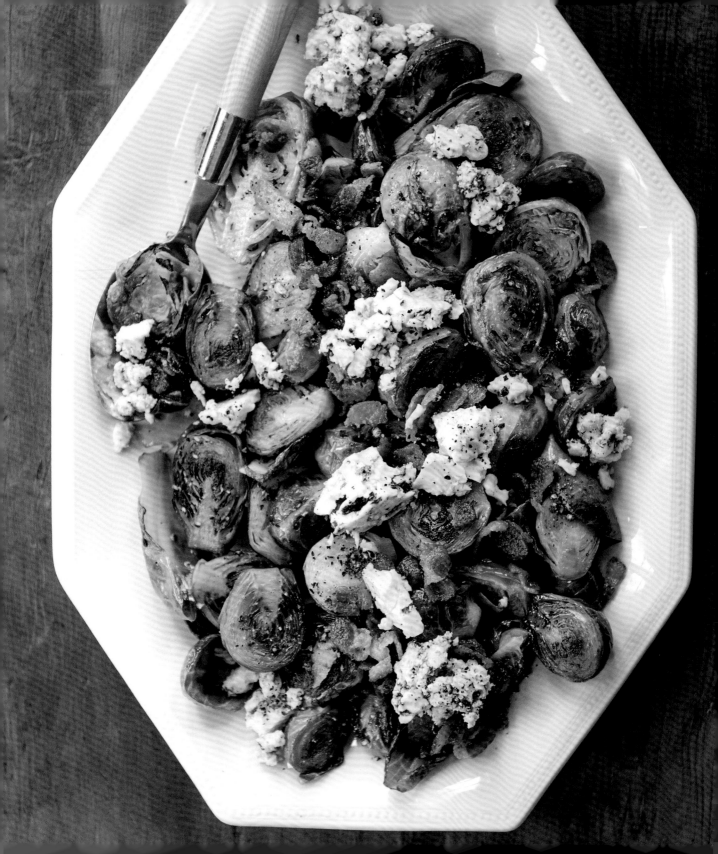

BRUSSELS SPROUTS WITH BACON & BLUE CHEESE

Give your Brussels sprouts the royal treatment by roasting them with bacon and then loading them with creamy crumbled blue cheese. In my experience, even the pickiest eaters can't resist this savory side.

SERVINGS: **4**   PREP TIME: **5 MINUTES**   COOK TIME: **20 MINUTES**

4 bacon slices, chopped

1 pound Brussels sprouts, trimmed and halved

Freshly ground black pepper

¼ cup crumbled blue cheese

IN a large cast-iron skillet, cook the bacon over medium-high heat, stirring occasionally, until crisp, 6 to 8 minutes. Using a slotted spoon, transfer the bacon to a paper towel–lined bowl and remove all but 1 tablespoon of the bacon fat from the skillet.

ADD the Brussels sprouts to the skillet, cut-side down. Cook, flipping occasionally, until the sprouts become golden and tender, about 10 minutes. Season with pepper. Return the bacon to the skillet and cook, stirring, for 2 minutes more.

TRANSFER the Brussels sprouts to a serving dish and top with the blue cheese. Serve immediately.

mix it up

Add 2 tablespoons maple syrup to the sprouts when you return the bacon back to the pan. Instead of blue cheese, top them with ½ cup toasted pecans.

GARLIC-THYME MUSHROOMS

VEGETARIAN
WHEAT-FREE
PESCATARIAN

If you're searching for the perfect side, I've got three words for you: Garlic. Thyme. Mushrooms. Sautéed in just a little butter, this trifecta of flavor never disappoints. This yummy dish would be the perfect accompaniment to the Easy-Peasy Risotto on page 165.

SERVINGS: **4**   PREP TIME: **5 MINUTES**   COOK TIME: **10 MINUTES**

2 tablespoons butter

1 pound cremini mushrooms, sliced

2 garlic cloves, minced

2 teaspoons fresh thyme leaves, plus a few sprigs for garnish

Salt and freshly ground black pepper

IN a large cast-iron skillet, melt the butter over medium-high heat. Add the mushrooms and cook, stirring often, until they release their moisture and begin to brown, 6 to 8 minutes. Add the garlic, thyme, and salt and pepper. Cook, stirring often, until the garlic is fragrant and the mushrooms are golden, about 2 minutes.

SERVE immediately, garnished with thyme springs, or store in the refrigerator for up to 3 days.

mix it up

While I use cremini mushrooms most often in my cooking, I also love to mix it up by combining a variety of fresh mushrooms like chanterelles, oyster, shiitakes, and chopped portobellos.

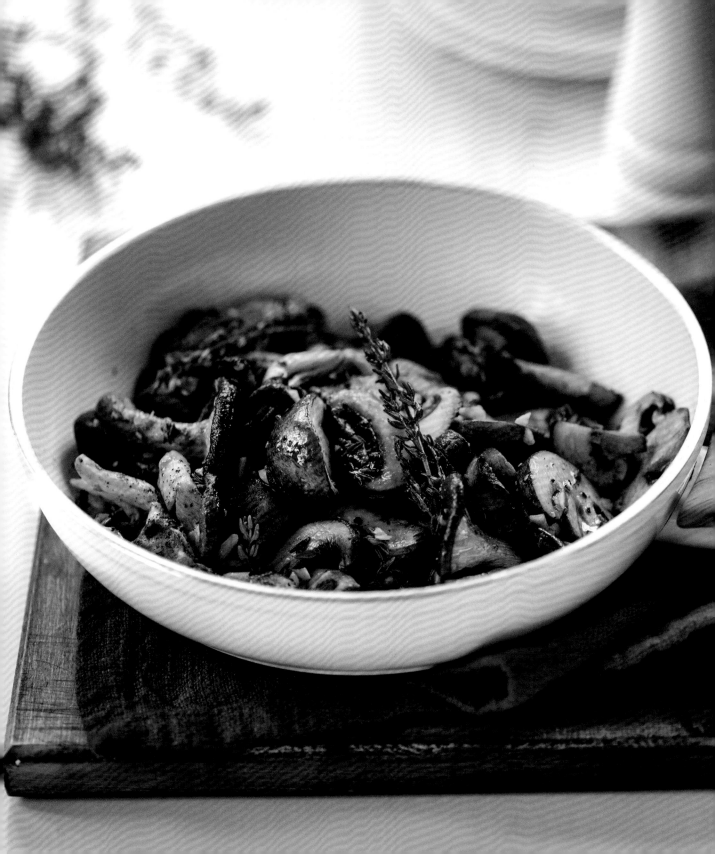

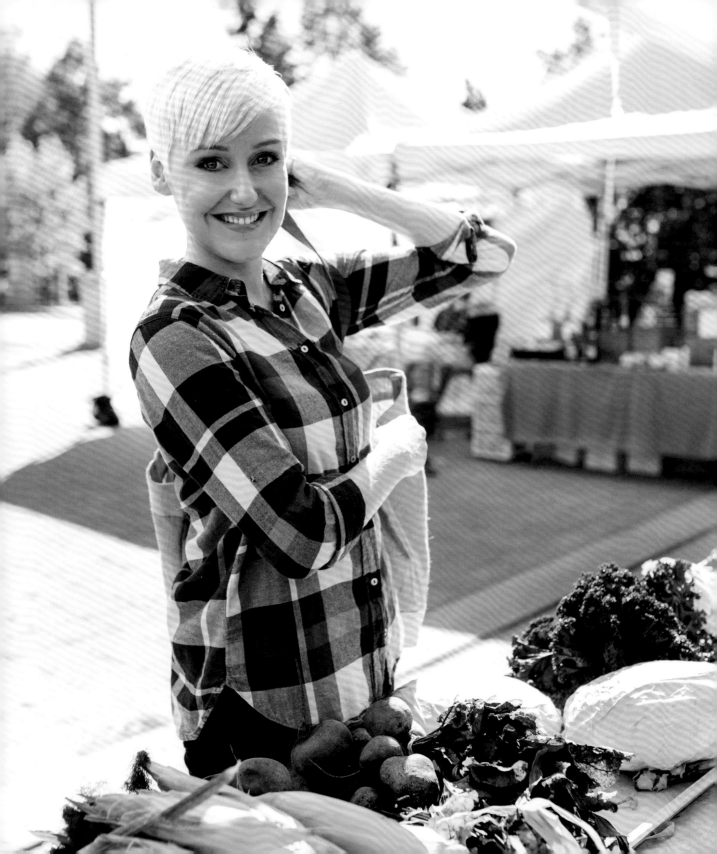

ROASTED ROOT VEGETABLES

VEGETARIAN
VEGAN
WHEAT-FREE
DAIRY-FREE
PESCATARIAN

Roasted Root Vegetables make such a satisfying side dish in the cool autumn and winter months. This warm, comforting combination of earthy veggies develops a natural sweetness when roasted that's perfectly balanced by a healthy splash of tangy red wine vinegar. I love pairing it with the Maple-Dijon Salmon on page 138 for a nourishing weeknight meal.

SERVINGS: **4**   PREP TIME: **10 MINUTES**   COOK TIME: **40 MINUTES**

---

2 medium red potatoes, diced

1 small rutabaga, peeled and diced

2 parsnips, peeled and diced

2 carrots, diced

1 red onion, cut into eighths

2 tablespoons extra-virgin olive oil

2 tablespoons red wine vinegar

1 teaspoon garlic powder

2 teaspoons fresh thyme leaves

Salt and freshly ground black pepper

PREHEAT the oven to 375°F.

ARRANGE the vegetables in an even layer in a large roasting pan. Add the olive oil, vinegar, garlic powder, thyme, and salt and pepper and toss until the vegetables are evenly coated.

ROAST the vegetables, tossing twice during the cooking time, for about 40 minutes, or until tender and golden on all sides.

SERVE immediately or store in the refrigerator for up to 4 days.

mix it up

You can mix up the flavors in this dish by adding different root vegetables. Try some peeled turnip, sweet potato, and/or beets.

CUCUMBER & WATERMELON SALAD

VEGETARIAN
WHEAT-FREE
PESCATARIAN

This refreshing salad is the most delicious way to beat the summer heat. It's crisp, sweet, and best served chilled, straight from the refrigerator. Its invigorating flavors make it great for serving at a BBQ or picnic. Plus, it's a perfect recipe for serving a crowd, since it's so easy to make.

SERVINGS: **4**   PREP TIME: **10 MINUTES**

---

2 tablespoons fresh lime juice

1 tablespoon honey

4 cups cubed watermelon

1 English cucumber, seeded and thinly sliced

¼ cup crumbled feta cheese

8 to 10 fresh mint leaves

IN a small bowl, whisk together the lime juice and honey until well combined.

IN a serving bowl, combine the watermelon and cucumber. Pour over the dressing and toss until everything is coated. Top with the feta and fresh mint. Refrigerate for 20 minutes before serving.

SERVE immediately, straight from the fridge, or store in the fridge for up to 2 days.

simple swaps

Swap out the fresh mint for summery fresh basil instead.

mix it up

To switch things up, skip the feta cheese and add ½ cup fresh blueberries instead.

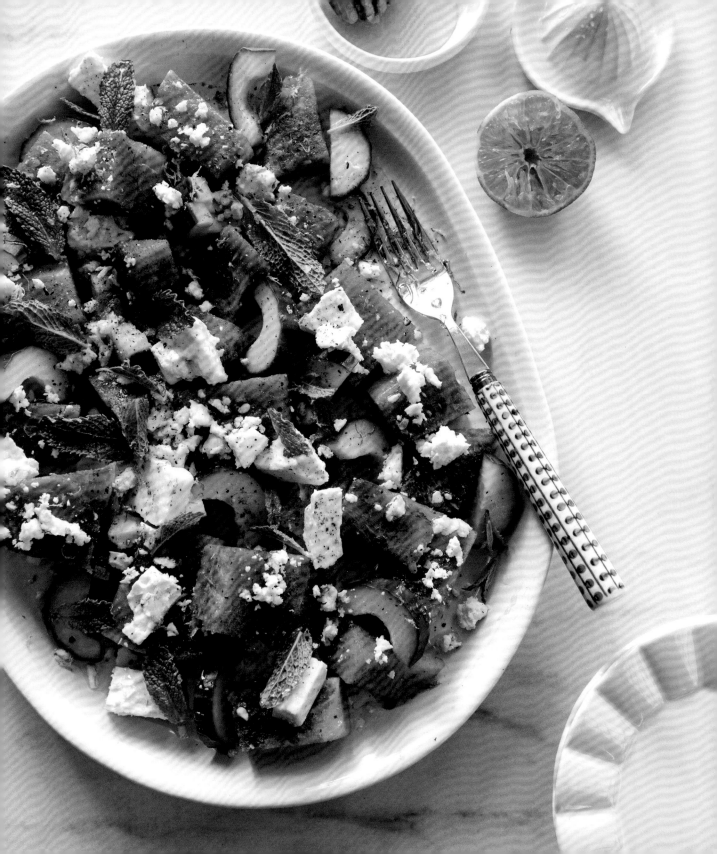

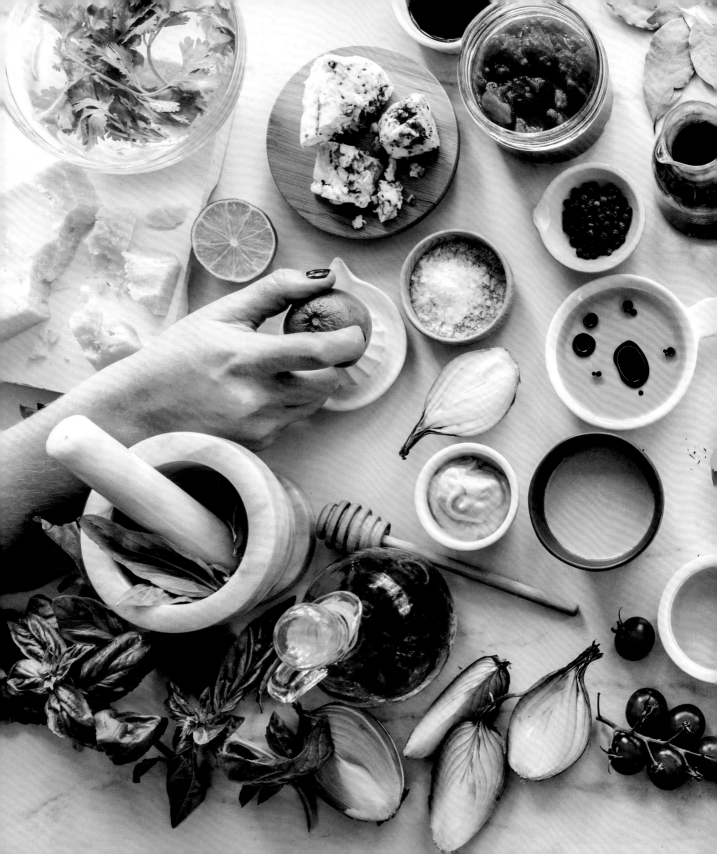

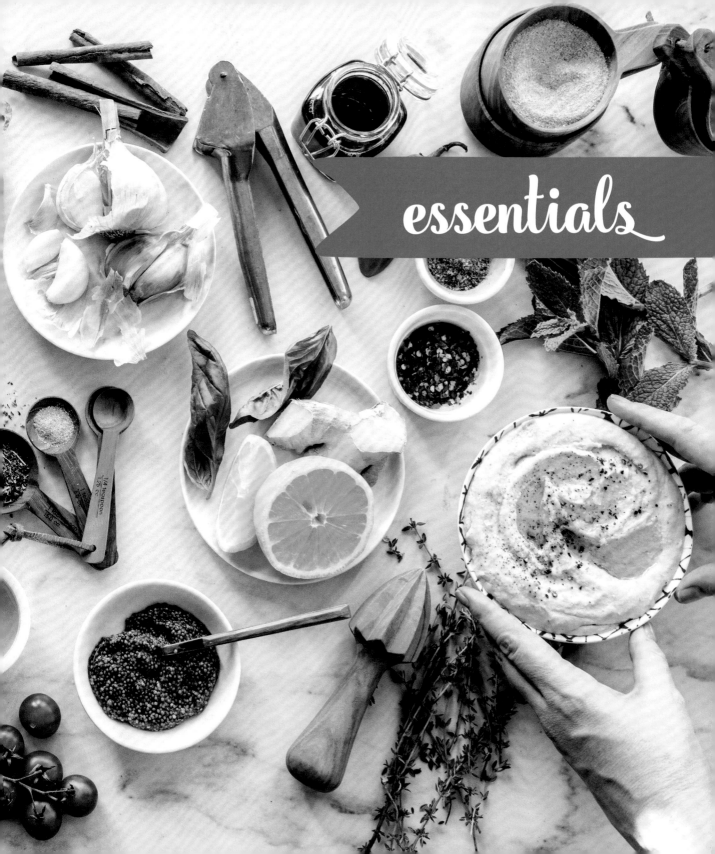

essentials

VEGETABLE BROTH

VEGETARIAN

VEGAN

WHEAT-FREE

DAIRY-FREE

PESCATARIAN

Broth is one of those staples that I can never have enough of, so much so that it tops my list of essentials. Homemade broth is surprisingly easy to make and can be so much more flavorful than the store-bought stuff. In addition, making your own broth allows you to control how much salt is added—bonus. I like to make broth during my Sunday meal prep. Once it's ready, I portion it into containers and store them in the freezer so I always have some on hand.

MAKES: **10 TO 12 CUPS**   PREP TIME: **5 MINUTES**   COOK TIME: **1 HOUR 30 MINUTES**

---

3 yellow onions, coarsely chopped

5 celery stalks, coarsely chopped

3 medium carrots, coarsely chopped

1 garlic head, cut in half crosswise to expose the cloves

10 fresh parsley sprigs

4 fresh thyme sprigs

2 teaspoons whole black peppercorns

Salt

PUT all the ingredients in a large Dutch oven or soup pot. Add enough water to completely submerge the ingredients (3 to 4 quarts should be enough). Bring the water to a boil over high heat, then reduce the heat to medium-low, cover, and simmer until the broth is golden and the flavors have concentrated, 1 hour 30 minutes to 2 hours. Check the seasoning at this point and add more salt if necessary.

USE a large slotted spoon or tongs to carefully remove and discard the solids. Place a sieve lined with cheesecloth over a large heatproof bowl and strain the broth through it. Let cool completely.

TRANSFER the cooled broth to airtight containers and store in the refrigerator for up to 4 days or in the freezer for up to 6 months.

(continued)

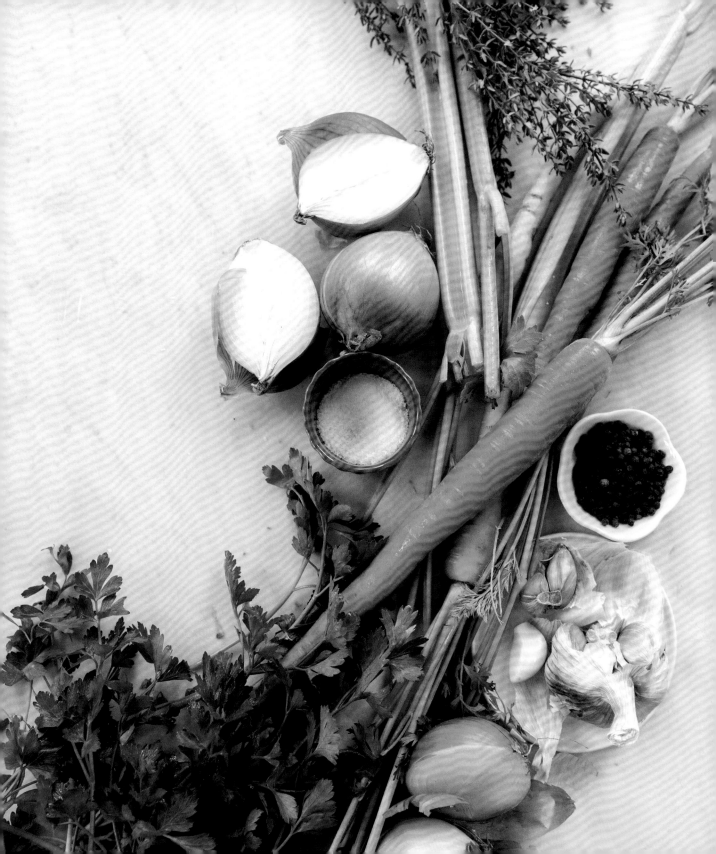

(Vegetable Broth continued)

mix it up

MUSHROOM BROTH

Add 3 cups chopped mixed mushrooms—cremini, white button, shiitake, or oyster mushrooms all work well—and 2 tablespoons soy sauce or tamari for more flavor.

SEAFOOD BROTH

Add 3 cups uncooked shrimp shells (I collect my shrimp shells over time and freeze them until I have enough for broth), 2 tablespoons tomato paste, and ½ cup white wine for more flavor.

CHICKEN BROTH

Add 1 (3- to 4-pound) whole chicken. Simmer until the chicken is completely cooked through, about 2 hours. Once the broth is ready, remove the cooked chicken and carve the cooked meat. I like to shred it and use it in recipes throughout the week. The cooked chicken can be stored in the refrigerator for up to 3 days or in the freezer for up to 3 months.

broth tips

1. You don't have to worry about peeling your onion, carrots, or garlic. The skins and peels can go right into the pot. Just give everything a thorough rinse before adding it.

2. I save my produce scraps—vegetable peels, onion skins, pepper cores, mushroom stems, broccoli stalks—throughout the week and store them in the freezer. When it's time to make broth, I add them all to the pot. It's a great way to get more from your produce.

3. To make the broth even more flavorful, gently roast the onions, carrots, celery, and garlic on a baking sheet at 350°F for 20 to 25 minutes before adding them to the soup pot.

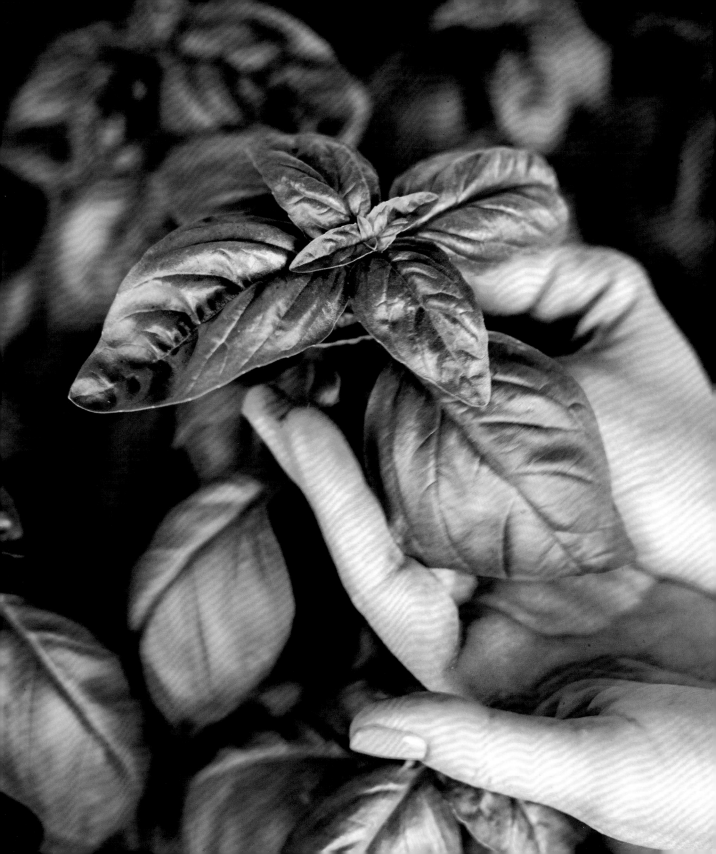

TOMATO SAUCE

VEGETARIAN
VEGAN
WHEAT-FREE
DAIRY-FREE
PESCATARIAN

It should be said that "tomato sauce" means different things to different people. Some people call this "marinara sauce," while others would say it's "pasta sauce." All I know is that this version is incredibly versatile, really flavorful, and so easy to make. I like to use it in all kinds of tasty recipes, which is why I always make a double or triple batch and then freeze the excess so it's always on hand.

SERVINGS: **8** PREP TIME: **5 MINUTES** COOK TIME: **25 MINUTES**

---

1 tablespoon extra-virgin olive oil

1 medium yellow onion, finely diced

5 garlic cloves, minced

2 (28-ounce) cans whole plum tomatoes, undrained

6 chopped fresh basil leaves

½ teaspoon dried oregano

1 dried bay leaf

Salt and freshly ground black pepper

IN a Dutch oven or large saucepan, heat the olive oil over medium-high heat. Add the onion and cook, stirring, until softened, about 4 minutes. Add the garlic and cook, stirring, for 1 minute. Add the tomatoes with their juices, the basil, oregano, and the bay leaf. Using the back of a wooden spoon, break up the tomatoes. Bring the mixture to a boil, then reduce the heat to medium-low and simmer until the flavors concentrate and the sauce thickens, about 20 minutes. Remove and discard the bay leaf and season with salt and pepper.

LEAVE the sauce a little chunky or, if you prefer, puree the sauce directly in the pot using an immersion blender to create a smoother sauce. (Alternatively, working in batches, carefully transfer the sauce to a standing blender and blend to your preferred consistency—be careful to let the liquid cool partially first when blending hot liquids.)

ENJOY immediately, or let cool completely and store in the refrigerator for up to 4 days or in the freezer for up to 6 months.

mix it up

This is a very basic recipe, but you can always jazz it up for even more great flavor.

- With your onion, add 1 finely chopped medium carrot and 2 finely chopped celery stalks.
- Try adding 2 fresh thyme sprigs with the other herbs.
- Finish the sauce by stirring in ⅓ cup freshly grated Parmesan cheese for a very rich, savory flavor.

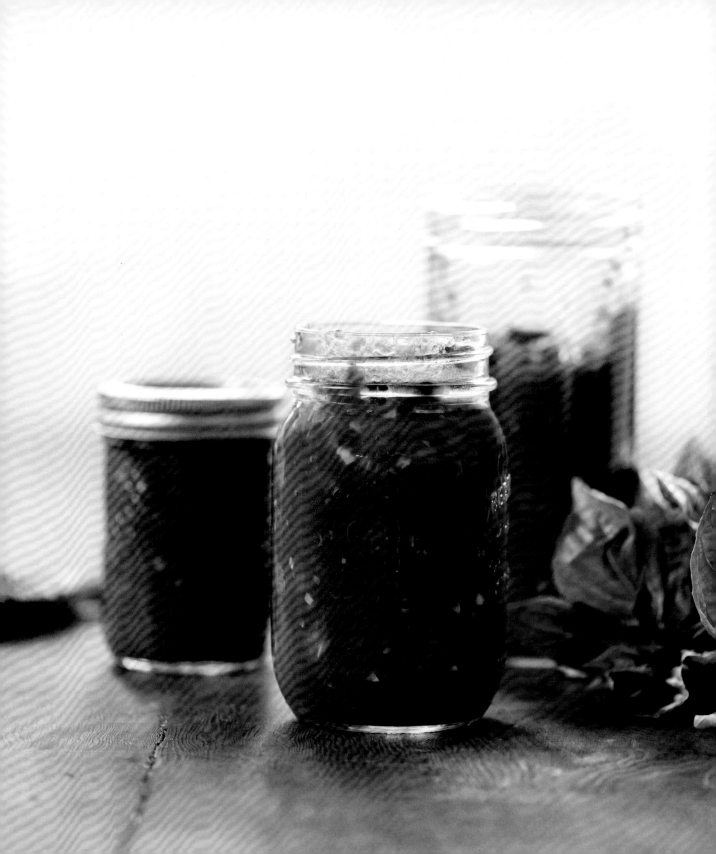

PESTO SAUCE

VEGETARIAN

VEGAN

WHEAT-FREE

DAIRY-FREE

PESCATARIAN

Pesto Sauce packs a major flavor punch thanks to its big, bold-tasting ingredients like fresh basil, garlic, and lots of Parmesan cheese. Store-bought pesto is fine, but nothing beats homemade, especially in the summer months when basil is at its most abundant. This delicious sauce can be enjoyed immediately over pasta or used in tasty recipes like the Caprese Chicken Quesadillas on page 120.

SERVINGS: **8**   PREP TIME: **5 MINUTES**

2 cups fresh basil leaves

2 garlic cloves, minced

¼ cup pine nuts

1 tablespoon fresh lemon juice

½ cup extra-virgin olive oil

¼ cup freshly grated
   Parmesan cheese

Salt and freshly ground black
   pepper

COMBINE the basil, garlic, pine nuts, and lemon juice in a food processor. Pulse for 30 seconds. With the motor running, slowly drizzle in the olive oil and process until the pesto is smooth.

TRANSFER to a bowl and add the Parmesan. Season with salt and pepper and stir well.

ENJOY immediately with pasta or in other recipes or store in the refrigerator for up to 5 days. It's a good idea to add a thin layer of olive oil on top of the sauce before refrigerating it to prevent oxidization.

simple swaps

- Try swapping out the pine nuts for ¼ cup toasted walnuts for a slightly different flavor. Keep in mind that this will make the pesto oxidize more quickly.
- Instead of using fresh garlic, add 3 roasted garlic cloves for a slightly sweeter, mellower flavor.
- Bump up the nutrition by swapping out 1 cup of the basil for 1 cup baby spinach or 1 cup baby kale.

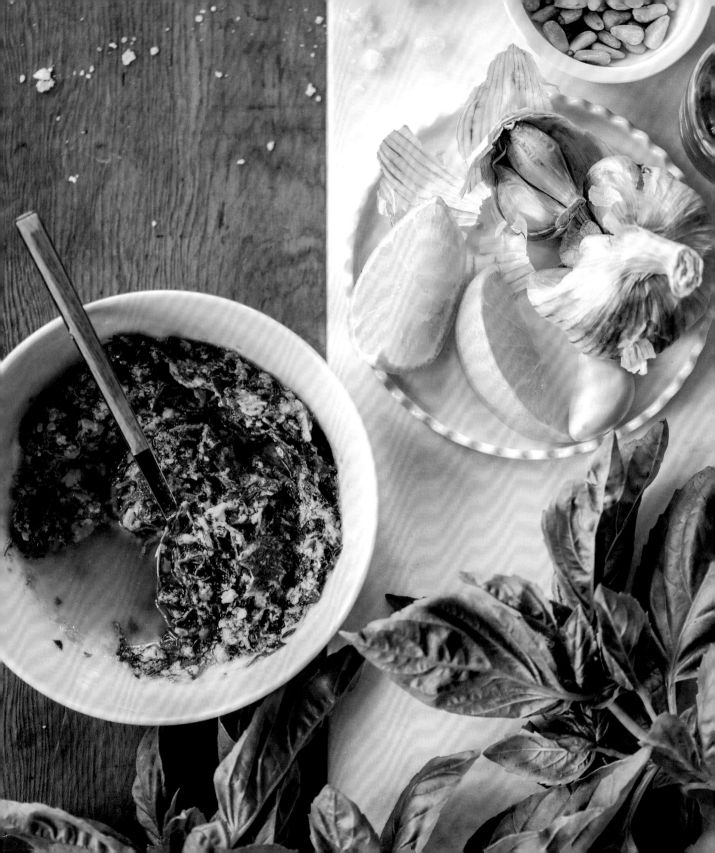

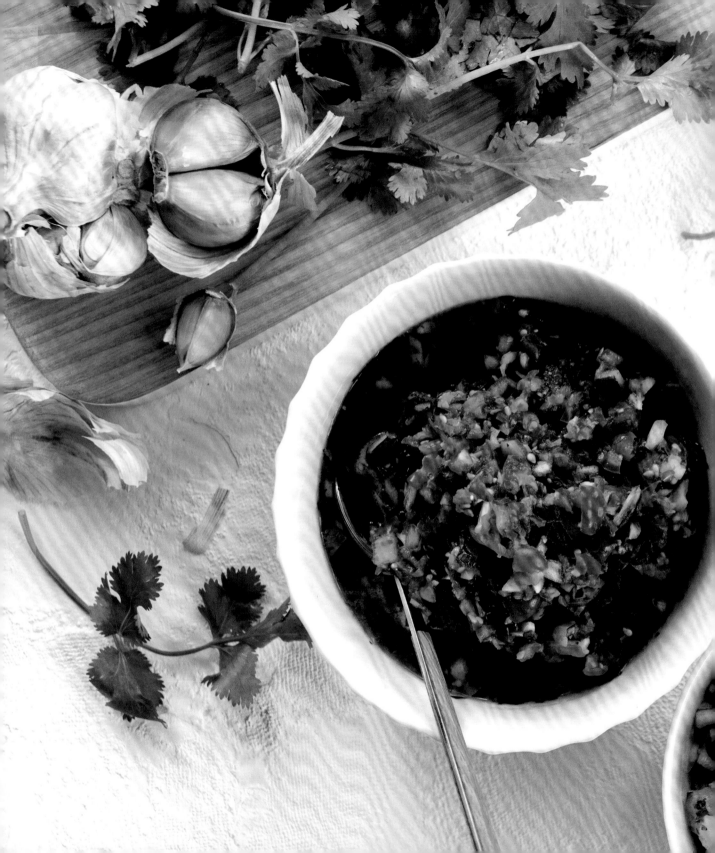

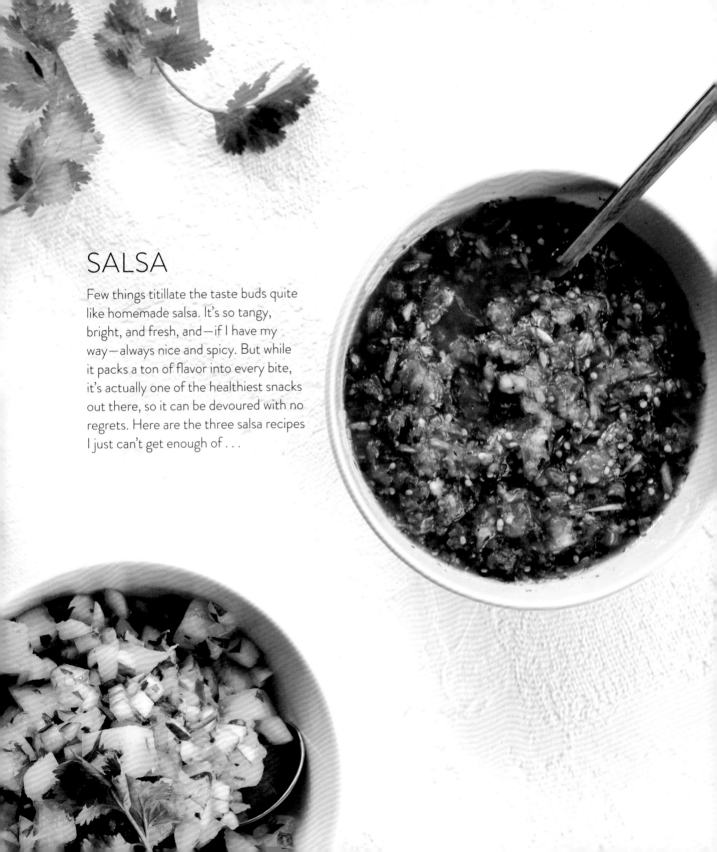

SALSA

Few things titillate the taste buds quite like homemade salsa. It's so tangy, bright, and fresh, and—if I have my way—always nice and spicy. But while it packs a ton of flavor into every bite, it's actually one of the healthiest snacks out there, so it can be devoured with no regrets. Here are the three salsa recipes I just can't get enough of . . .

SALSA FRESCA

SERVINGS: **4**   PREP TIME: **5 MINUTES**

1 pound cherry tomatoes

1 small red onion, finely diced

¼ cup fresh cilantro leaves

1 jalapeño, seeded and minced (optional)

1 garlic clove, minced

1 tablespoon red wine vinegar

1 tablespoon extra-virgin olive oil

Grated zest and juice of 1 lime

Salt and freshly ground black pepper

PUT the tomatoes in a food processor and gently pulse until they start to break down. Add the onion, cilantro, jalapeño (if using), garlic, vinegar, olive oil, lime zest, and lime juice. Pulse until you reach the desired consistency; it can be enjoyed chunkier or very smooth—up to you. Season with salt and pepper.

ENJOY immediately or store in the refrigerator for up to 5 days.

simple swaps

If you're not a fan of cilantro, swap in some fresh basil or parsley instead.

SALSA VERDE

SERVINGS: **4**   PREP TIME: **5 MINUTES**   COOK TIME: **10 MINUTES**

1 pound tomatillos, husked and rinsed

1 small white onion, quartered

1 jalapeño (optional)

¼ cup chopped fresh cilantro

2 garlic cloves, minced

Grated zest and juice of 1 lime

Salt and freshly ground black pepper

PREHEAT the broiler.

ARRANGE the tomatillos, onion, and jalapeño (if using) on a baking sheet. Broil, flipping once, for about 10 minutes, or until they are nicely charred.

CAREFULLY transfer the charred vegetables to a food processor. Add the cilantro, garlic, lime zest, and lime juice and pulse until the salsa reaches your desired consistency. Season with salt and pepper.

SERVE immediately or store in the refrigerator for up to 5 days.

simple swaps

For a smokier flavor, instead of using a jalapeño in this recipe, try adding 1 canned chipotle pepper in adobo sauce. Don't roast it with the tomatillos and onion; just add it to the food processor while blending.

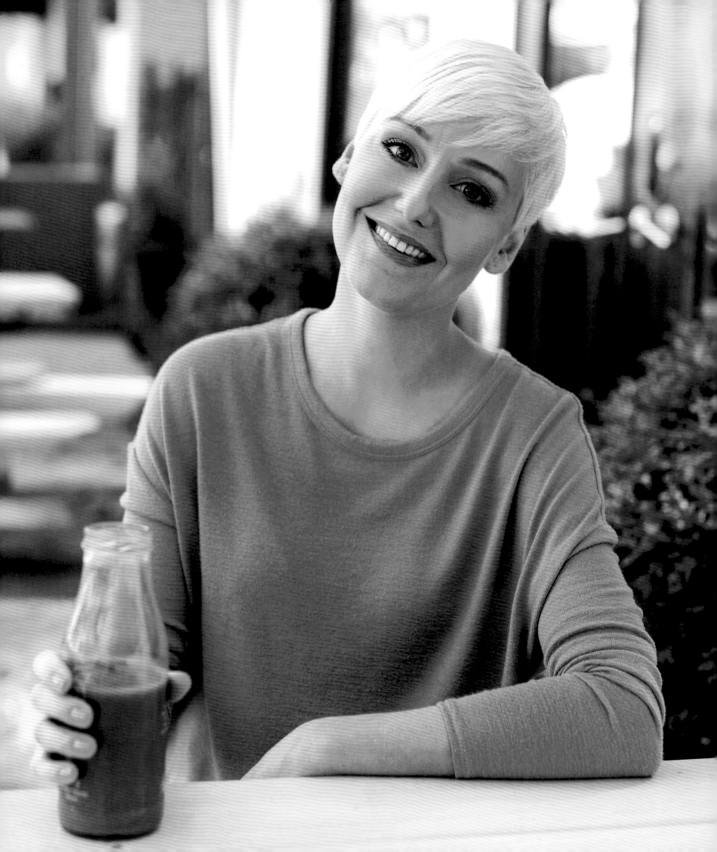

PINEAPPLE SALSA

SERVINGS: **4**   PREP TIME: **5 MINUTES**

½ pineapple, cored and finely diced

½ small red onion, finely diced

¼ cup chopped fresh cilantro

½ jalapeño, seeded and minced (optional)

Grated zest and juice of 1 lime

Salt and freshly ground black pepper

IN a medium bowl, combine the pineapple, red onion, cilantro, jalapeño (if using), lime zest, and lime juice. Season with salt and pepper and mix well.

SERVE immediately or store in the refrigerator for up to 4 days.

simple swaps

Instead of pineapple, use 2 cups finely diced ripe mango for a slightly different flavor.

CLASSIC GUACAMOLE

Is there anyone out there who doesn't love guacamole? It's cool and refreshing but still rich and creamy. It's tart, spicy, smooth, fresh . . . I could go on and on. But if you've only ever had store-bought guacamole, you are really missing out, because absolutely nothing compares to homemade, and you won't believe just how easy it is to get your guac on.

SERVINGS: **4**   PREP TIME: **5 MINUTES**

3 ripe avocados

Grated zest and juice of 1 lime

¼ red onion, finely diced

½ jalapeño, seeded and minced (optional)

1 garlic clove, minced

¼ cup chopped fresh cilantro

¼ teaspoon ground cumin

Salt and freshly ground black pepper

IN a large bowl, use a potato masher or fork to mash the avocados with the lime zest and juice. You can make the avocado very smooth or leave it slightly chunky; it's totally a matter of preference.

STIR in the onion, jalapeño (if using), garlic, cilantro, and cumin. Season with salt and pepper.

ENJOY immediately or store in the refrigerator for up to 3 days. To prevent the guacamole from browning, cover the surface with ¼ inch of water. Before eating it, simply pour off the water and give it a stir.

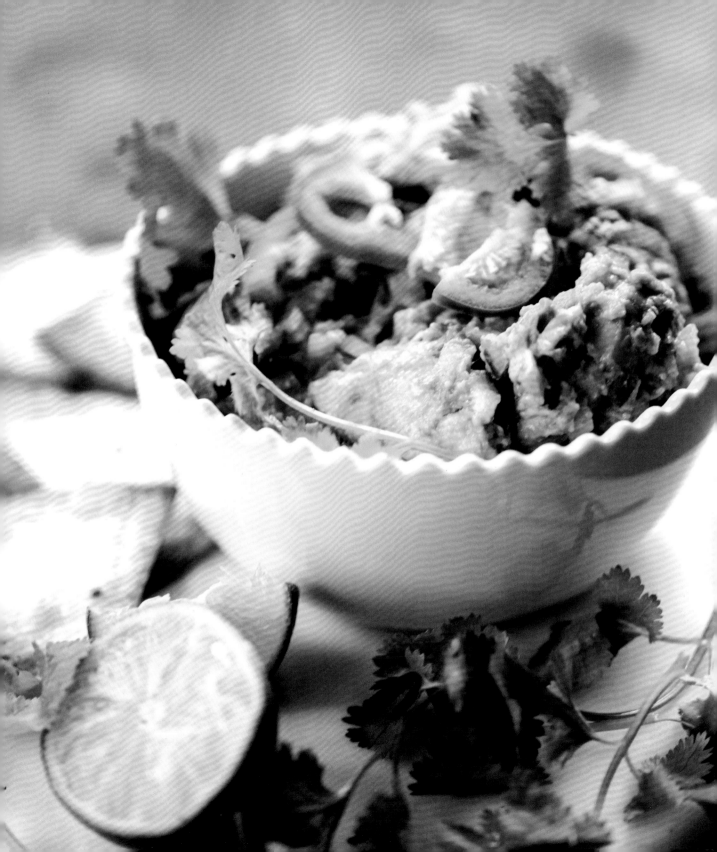

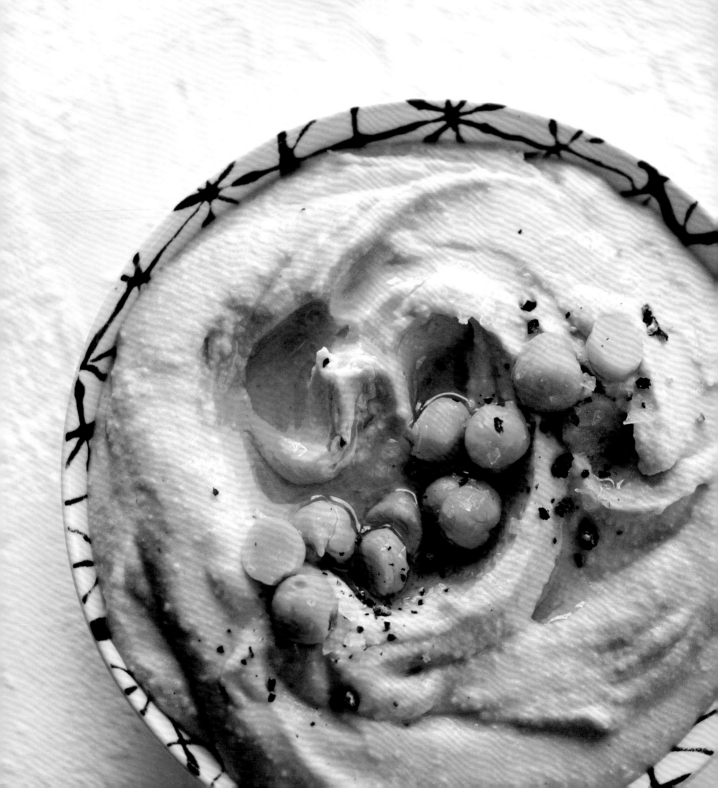

CLASSIC HUMMUS

Smooth, creamy, garlicky hummus is simply one of the best snacks out there. It's loaded with fiber and protein, so it's very satiating and is a really versatile ingredient that can be added to pastas, soups, or salads or enjoyed all on its own. And once you've got the basic recipe down, there are dozens of ways to dress it up.

SERVINGS: **4**   PREP TIME: **5 MINUTES**

1 (15-ounce) can chickpeas, drained and rinsed (save some for serving, if desired)

3 garlic cloves, minced

2 tablespoons fresh lemon juice

1 tablespoon tahini paste

Salt and freshly ground black pepper

¼ cup extra-virgin olive oil, plus more for serving

IN a food processor, combine the chickpeas, garlic, lemon juice, tahini, and salt and pepper. Process until the mixture begins to become smooth. With the motor running, slowly drizzle in the olive oil and process until the hummus is completely smooth and reaches your desired consistency.

SERVE immediately with a drizzle of olive oil, some whole chickpeas, if desired, and salt and pepper, or store in the refrigerator for up to 5 days.

mix it up

DILL PICKLE HUMMUS
Blend in ¼ cup chopped dill pickles, 2 tablespoons dill pickle brine (from the jar), and 2 tablespoons chopped fresh dill.

ROASTED BEET HUMMUS
Blend in ½ cup chopped roasted beets.

GREEN GODDESS HUMMUS
Blend in ¼ cup chopped fresh parsley, 2 tablespoons chopped fresh chives, and 2 tablespoons chopped fresh tarragon.

TZATZIKI SAUCE

Cool and refreshing with a tangy twist, Tzatziki Sauce is my dip of choice for fresh veggies and a great addition to any Mediterranean-inspired dish. You can purchase tzatziki sauce premade at most supermarkets, but once you discover how easy it is to make your own, you'll probably never go back.

VEGETARIAN
WHEAT-FREE
PESCATARIAN

SERVINGS: **4**   PREP TIME: **10 MINUTES**

---

1 English cucumber, peeled and seeded

1 cup plain Greek yogurt

2 garlic cloves, grated

Grated zest and juice of ½ lemon

2 tablespoons chopped fresh dill

Salt and freshly ground black pepper

GRATE the cucumber, then transfer it to a clean kitchen towel, gather the sides, and twist to squeeze the excess liquid from it.

IN a medium bowl, combine the grated cucumber, yogurt, garlic, lemon zest, lemon juice, and dill. Stir well and season with salt and pepper.

ENJOY immediately or store in the refrigerator for up to 4 days.

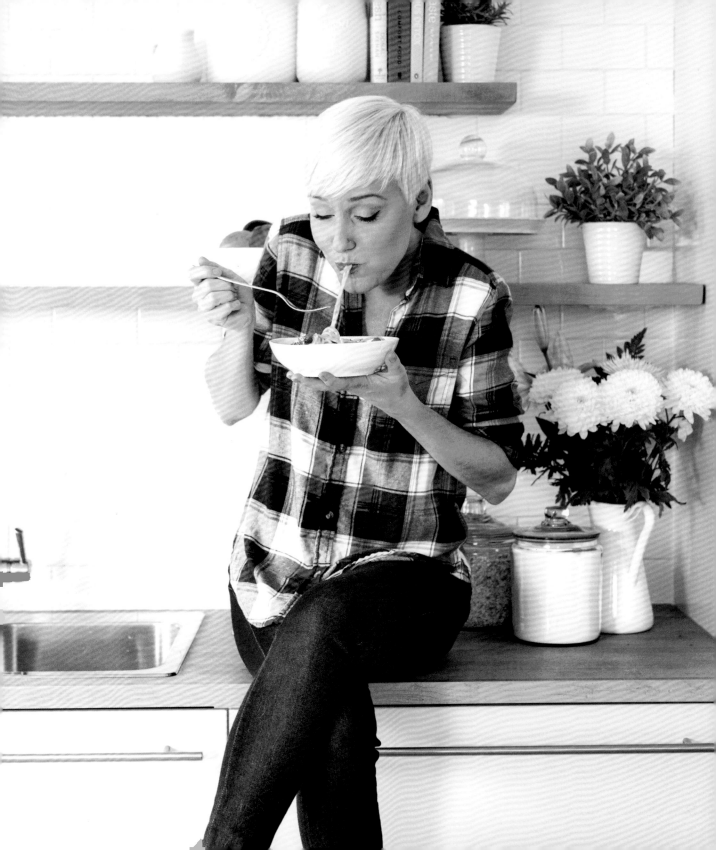

CLASSIC DRESSINGS

Store-bought dressings can be loaded with unnecessary added salt, sugar, and fat, so homemade is definitely the healthier way to go. These classic dressing recipes are fresh and flavorful, and use simple ingredients you probably already have in your fridge and pantry.

MAKES: **ABOUT ½ CUP**   PREP TIME: **5 MINUTES**

WHITE WINE VINAIGRETTE

¼ cup extra-virgin olive oil

3 tablespoons white wine vinegar

1 tablespoon fresh lemon juice

1 tablespoon honey

1 teaspoon Dijon mustard

Salt and freshly ground black pepper

VEGETARIAN
WHEAT-FREE
DAIRY-FREE
PESCATARIAN

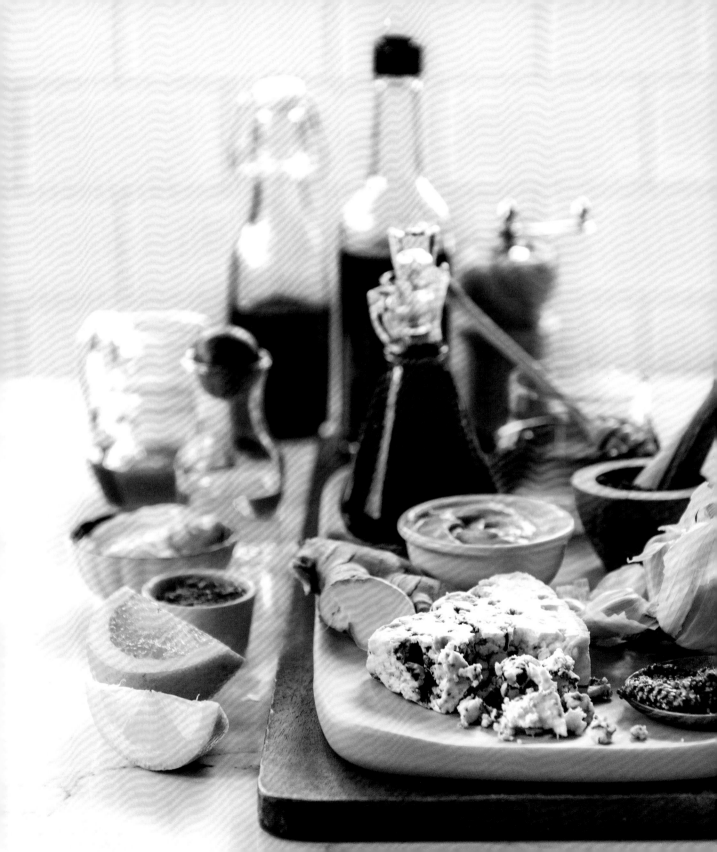

BALSAMIC VINAIGRETTE

¼ cup extra-virgin olive oil

3 tablespoons balsamic vinegar

1 teaspoon Dijon mustard

1 garlic clove, grated

Salt and freshly ground black pepper

ITALIAN DRESSING

¼ cup extra-virgin olive oil

3 tablespoons red wine vinegar

1 teaspoon Italian Seasoning (page 230)

1 teaspoon Dijon mustard

1 garlic clove, grated

Salt and freshly ground black pepper

BLUE CHEESE DRESSING

¼ cup plain yogurt

2 tablespoons mayonnaise

2 tablespoons crumbled blue cheese

½ teaspoon Worcestershire sauce

Salt and freshly ground black pepper

ASIAN GINGER DRESSING

¼ cup canola oil

3 tablespoons rice vinegar

1 tablespoon soy sauce

1 tablespoon honey

1 garlic clove, grated

½ teaspoon grated fresh ginger

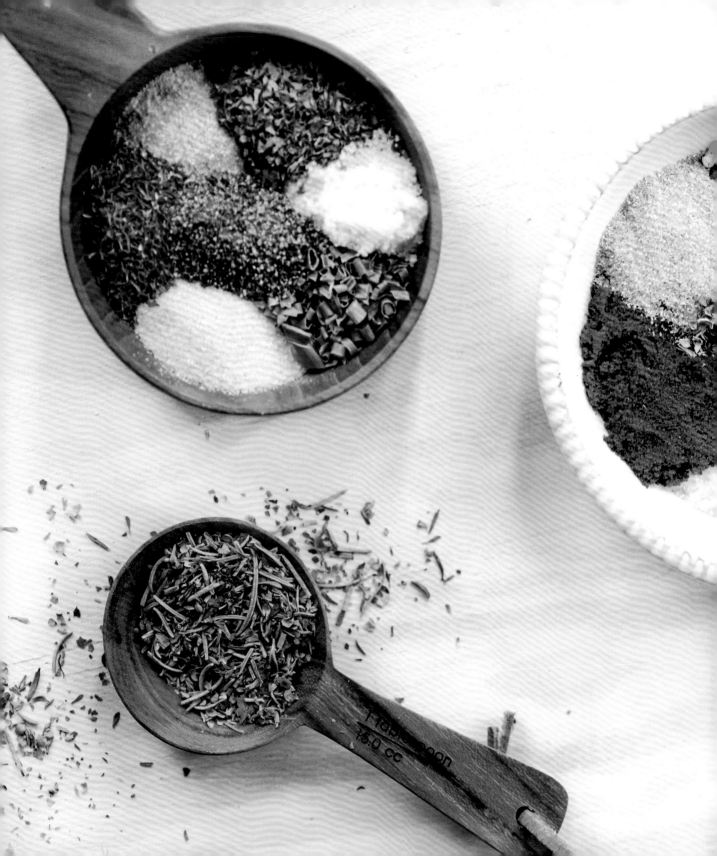

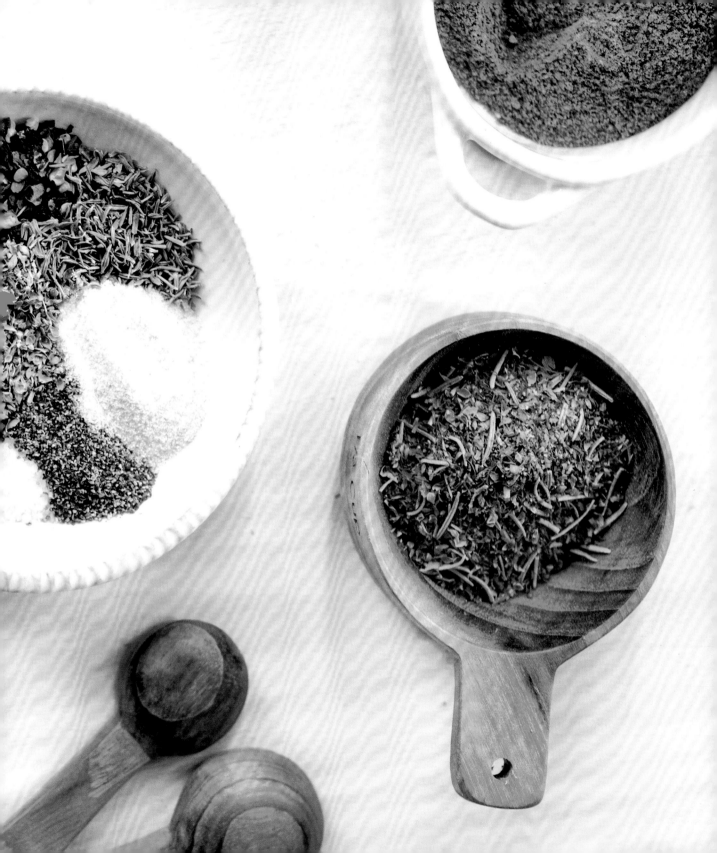

SPICE BLENDS

The spice aisle in your supermarket is likely packed with countless seasoning blends, but you might be surprised by how simple and affordable they are to make at home. Here are my five favorites, which I use constantly in my cooking. Feel free to adjust them to your own tastes. Just stir the ingredients together and then store the prepared blends in airtight containers for up to 6 months.

MAKES: **ABOUT ¾ CUP**   PREP TIME: **5 MINUTES**

VEGETARIAN
VEGAN
WHEAT-FREE
DAIRY-FREE
PESCATARIAN

GREEK SEASONING

2 tablespoons dried oregano

1 tablespoon dried basil

1 tablespoon dried thyme

1 tablespoon dried rosemary

1 tablespoon dried parsley

1 tablespoon dried dill

1 tablespoon onion powder

1 tablespoon garlic powder

1 tablespoon salt

1 tablespoon freshly ground black pepper

1 teaspoon ground cinnamon

1 teaspoon ground nutmeg

ITALIAN SEASONING

2 tablespoons dried basil

2 tablespoons dried oregano

1 tablespoon dried rosemary

1 tablespoon dried sage

1 tablespoon dried thyme

1 tablespoon dried parsley

1 tablespoon dried marjoram

1 tablespoon salt

1 tablespoon freshly ground black pepper

CAJUN SEASONING

¼ cup paprika

2 tablespoons garlic powder

2 tablespoons onion powder

1 tablespoon salt

1 tablespoon freshly ground black pepper

2 teaspoons dried oregano

2 teaspoons dried thyme

1 teaspoon cayenne pepper (optional)

1 teaspoon red pepper flakes (optional)

PUMPKIN PIE SPICE

⅓ cup ground cinnamon

¼ cup ground ginger

1 tablespoon ground allspice

1 tablespoon ground nutmeg

1 tablespoon ground cloves

RANCH SEASONING

3 tablespoons dried parsley

2 tablespoons garlic powder

2 tablespoons onion powder

1 tablespoon dried dill

1 tablespoon dried chives

1 tablespoon salt

1 tablespoon freshly ground black pepper

index

Note: Page references in *italics* indicate photographs.

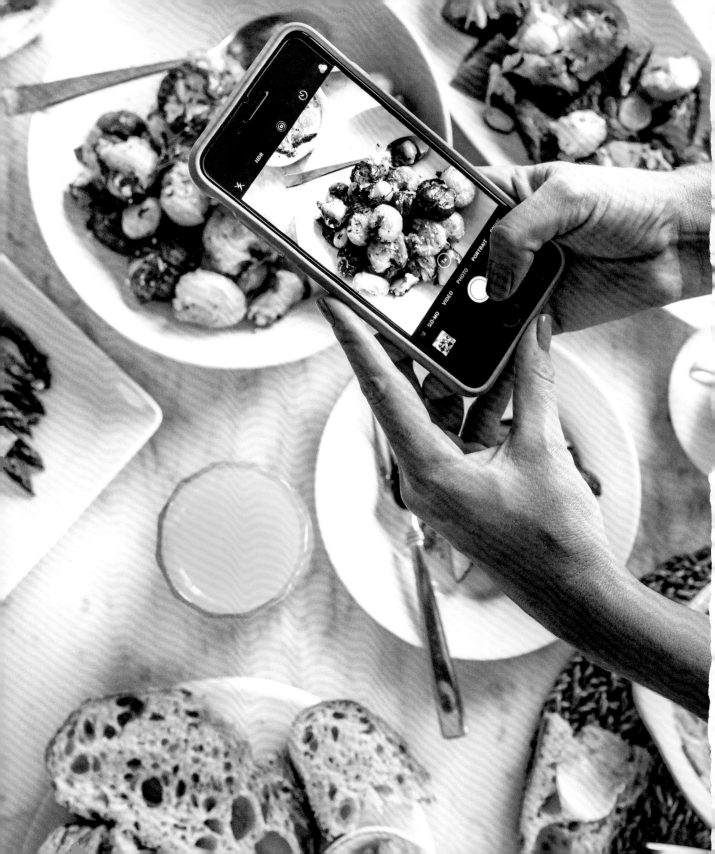